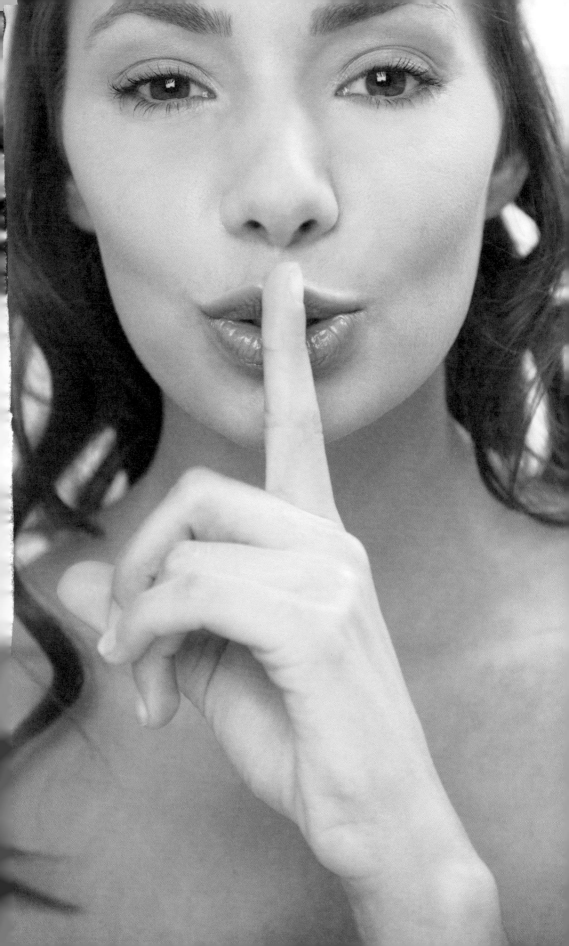

NICOLE BAILEY

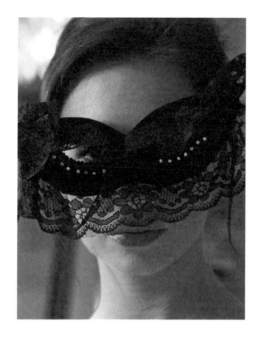

SEX
SECRETS

DUNCAN BAIRD PUBLISHERS

LONDON

SEX SECRETS
NICOLE BAILEY

Distributed in the USA and Canada by
Sterling Publishing Co., Inc.
387 Park Avenue South
New York, NY 10016-8810

This edition first published in the UK and USA in 2011 by
Duncan Baird Publishers Ltd
Sixth Floor, Castle House
75–76 Wells Street
London W1T 3QH

Managing Editor: Grace Cheetham
Editor: Dawn Bates
Managing Designer: Manisha Patel
Art Direction and Design: Emma and Tom Forge
Commissioned Photography: John Davis
Commissioned Illustrations: Susie Hogarth

Library of Congress Cataloging-in-Publication Data available

ISBN: 978-1-84483-923-0

10 9 8 7 6 5 4 3 2 1

Typeset in Conduit ITC
Color reproduction by Scanhouse, Malaysia
Printed in Singapore by Imago

For information about custom editions, special sales, premium and corporate purchases, please
contact Sterling Special Sales Department at 800-805-5489 or specialsales@sterlingpub.com.

PUBLISHER'S NOTE:
The Publisher, the author, and the photographer cannot accept any responsibility for any injuries or
damages incurred as a result of following the advice in this book, or of using any of the techniques
described or mentioned herein. If you suffer from any health problems or special conditions, it is
recommended that you consult your doctor before following any practice suggested in this book.
Some of the advice in this book involves the use of massage oil. However, do not use massage oil if
you are using a condom—the oil damages latex.

Outdoor sex, in places of free public access, is illegal in many jurisdictions, and anyone who chooses
to have sex outside, or to be less than fully clothed in public, should inform themselves of the
possible penalties (which in some countries are very severe) and be thoroughly aware of the risks.
Neither the publisher nor the author can take any responsibility for any legal action or other
unintended consequences resulting from following any of the advice or suggestions in this book.

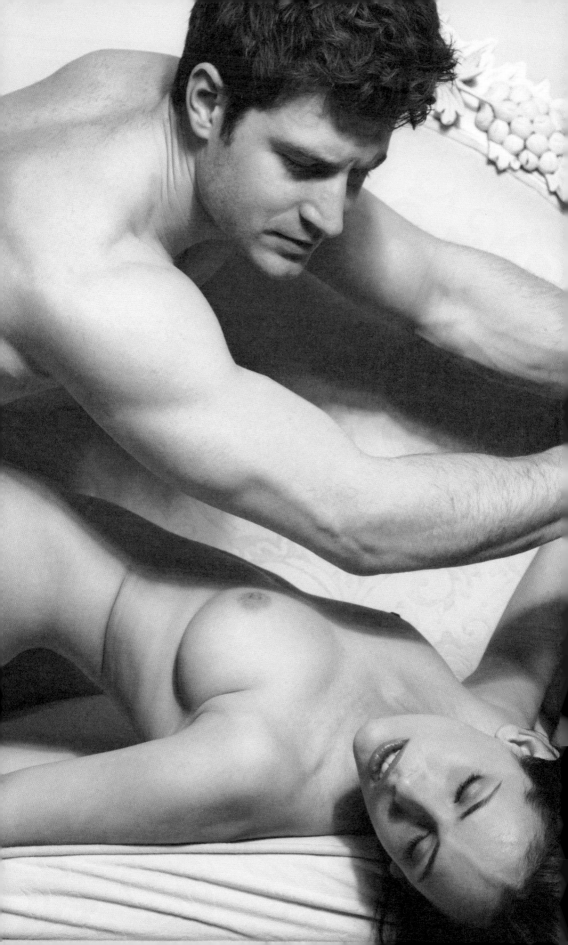

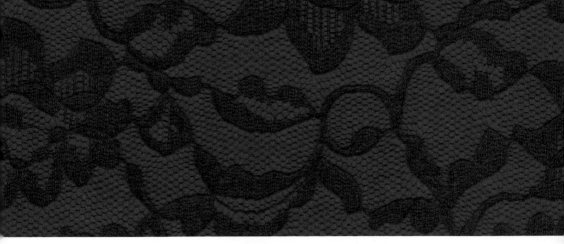

Contents

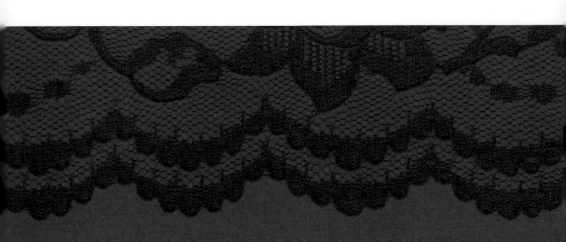

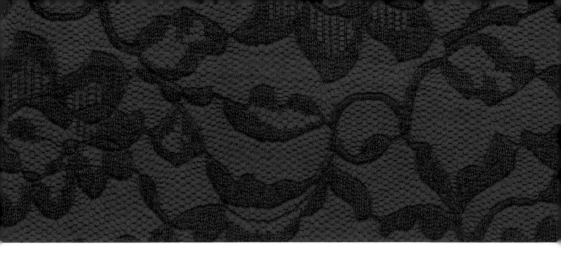

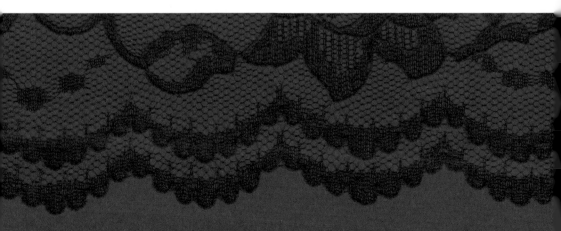

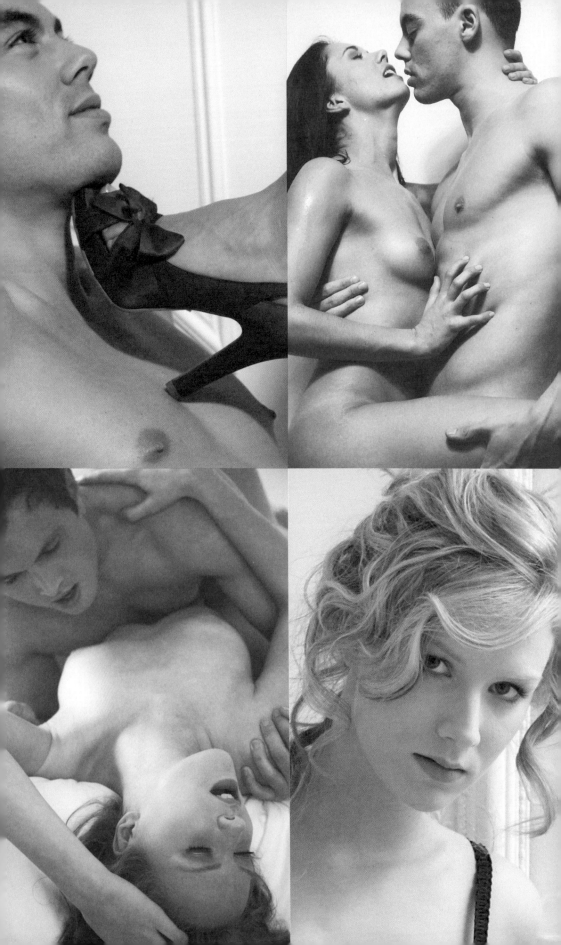

Introduction

I've noticed that whenever I get together with my female friends, over the course of an evening the conversation slowly but surely turns to sex. We share experiences from past and present, as well as fantasies about the future. I love these conversations with other women. As well as being fun, they're also liberating, enlightening and informative – I've learnt so much from them. This was one of my main inspirations for writing *Sex Secrets*: to share my own experiences and those of other women. After all there's something very valuable about being given a sex tip that's been personally tried and tested.

BE A CONFIDENT SEDUCTRESS

The first chapter is all about Seduction. As well as tips on how to flirt, talk dirty and take your clothes off, I've included dozens of secrets to build your sexual confidence. From my conversations I've realized that it's fairly common for women to rely on men to make the first move. A close friend of mine confessed that she had always played a very passive role until she found herself going out with a man who worked so hard he barely had time for a cuddle, let alone sex. She realized that, to tear him away from his desk, she needed to make a special effort. So she went all out to make herself the centre of attention. Her surprise discovery was that she really started to enjoy herself. My own experience backs this up – being the seductress makes me feel not just sexy, but powerful too. Plus men have told me that they appreciate sexual assertiveness because it allows them to sit back and relax a little.

My hope is that you'll find and enjoy your inner seductress. Sometimes seduction can be subtle: looks, touches, gestures and a flirtatious undercurrent that runs through your conversations. Other times it's big and brazen, like when you lure him into the bedroom and perform a mesmerizing striptease to music. Seduction techniques might seem as though they're all for his pleasure, but the truth is, you'll find them just as thrilling as he does.

HAVE DELICIOUS FOREPLAY

Chapter 2 is all about foreplay. Some people don't rate foreplay because they see it as the "boring bit" before the action. I disagree. For me foreplay is the fun and carefree part, where you get to play around, experiment and connect. I've included my favourite ways of doing this, from slow and sensual massage to red-hot oral sex techniques. And, because women tell me how much they appreciate the right kind of stimulation, I've shared the secrets of getting him to touch you the way you want. Plus there's a guide to all your internal hotspots (including some you probably didn't know you had). So whether you spend an hour on sensual stroking or five minutes on passionate oral sex, I hope you'll both be sizzling with arousal by the time you have sex.

ENJOY EXPLOSIVE ORGASMS

In Chapter 3, Orgasm, my mission is to make that climactic moment as enjoyable and intense as possible. It became clear to me when I started having sex that men and women come in different ways and at different speeds. For example, my partner always climaxed quickly through intercourse, whereas I didn't. I knew I needed techniques that would maximize both my pleasure and his. Fortunately, through experimenting and talking to other women, I discovered all sorts of exciting ways to slow my partner down or to intensify my own sensations. Plus, over time, I discovered how my body works and what sort of orgasms are possible (there are several types!). I've put all of these orgasm secrets and more into Chapter 4. You can also read some fascinating first-person confessions.

TREAT SEX AS AN ADVENTURE

I love being playful and daring in bed. Some of my most memorable evenings have happened when I've set out to experiment – which is why I've devoted the whole of Chapter 4 to sexual adventures. I've included my favourite games and naughty activities, plus those of other women. For example, how to play sex dares, make an erotic film or arouse each other with sexy power games. And if you have an "I-can't-do-that-moment", I hope that the sexual confessions and anecdotes will inspire you to leave your comfort zone. It's worth it!

Writing *Sex Secrets* has been great fun. I've really enjoyed looking back over all my sexual experiences and talking to other people about theirs. I hope you and your lover have a fantastic time trying out the techniques.

Nicole Bailey

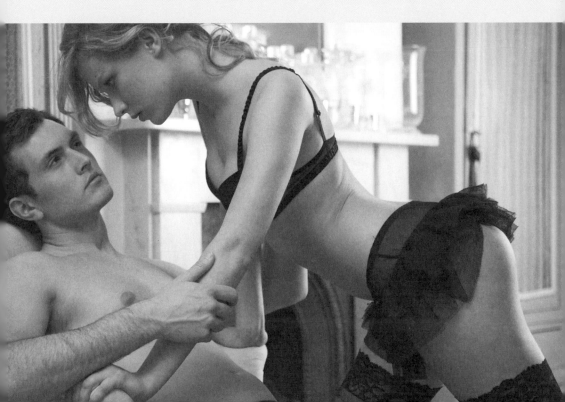

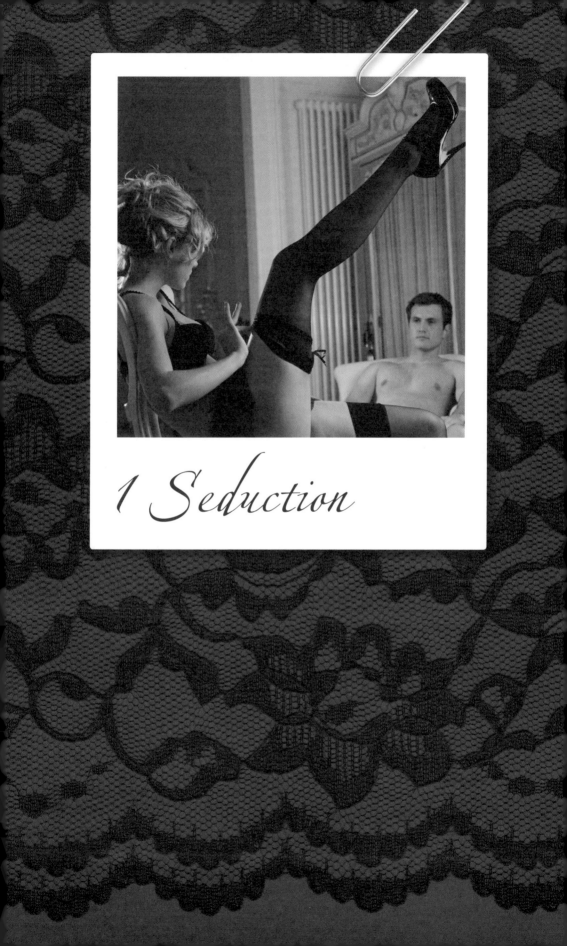

1 Seduction

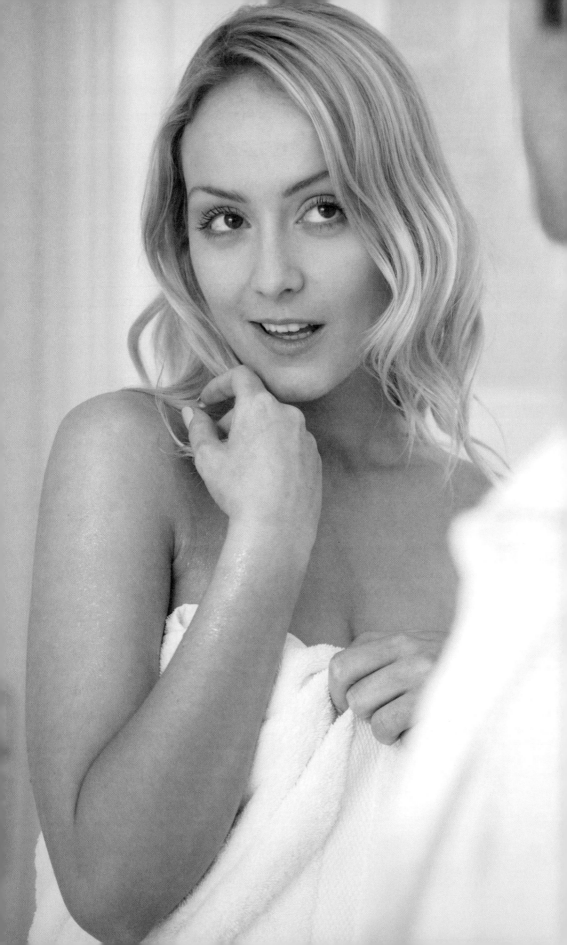

SET THE MOOD TO HOT

Some of my sexiest and most pleasurable nights have been those where I've held back from my lover at first, then slowly but surely built up a mood of erotic intensity. Close your eyes and imagine the scene: your lover is on his way over, you're dying to see him and the only thought on your mind is that first delicious kiss. It may be tempting to pounce on him as soon he walks in the door. Don't! Instead try this ...

Take a long, hot shower and greet him at the door wearing only a towel, your skin still glistening with moisture. Now invite him in and ask him to open that bottle of wine you've been chilling. Kiss him briefly on the lips, then wink and leave him to simmer for five minutes while you go off to change into something skimpy and provocative. Continue your hands-off approach as you share a glass of wine in the bedroom. Flirt with him, turning up the heat a degree at a time: move a little closer, hold his gaze a little longer and casually show off your sexiest assets. Make it subtle, though – give him the impression he's the one in control and making all the moves.

When he finally touches you, respond with slow sensuality rather than rampant desire. Pull back after each kiss, look into his eyes and tell him how good he tastes. Treat him like a gourmet meal you want to savour – even if he's trying to cut to the chase. If necessary, give him cooling-off time by popping to the bathroom. Prolong the anticipation for as long as possible.

Don't worry if this kind of seduction seems orchestrated – taking an active role can inflame your mood as much as half-an-hour of foreplay. You benefit and so does he.

BE ADVENTUROUS

Surprise is another great seduction tool. Treat sex as an opportunity to be really creative. Instead of following a formula of, say, stilettos, silk knickers and satin sheets, try an alternative approach, such as roleplay, reading erotica to each other or having sex outside of the bedroom.

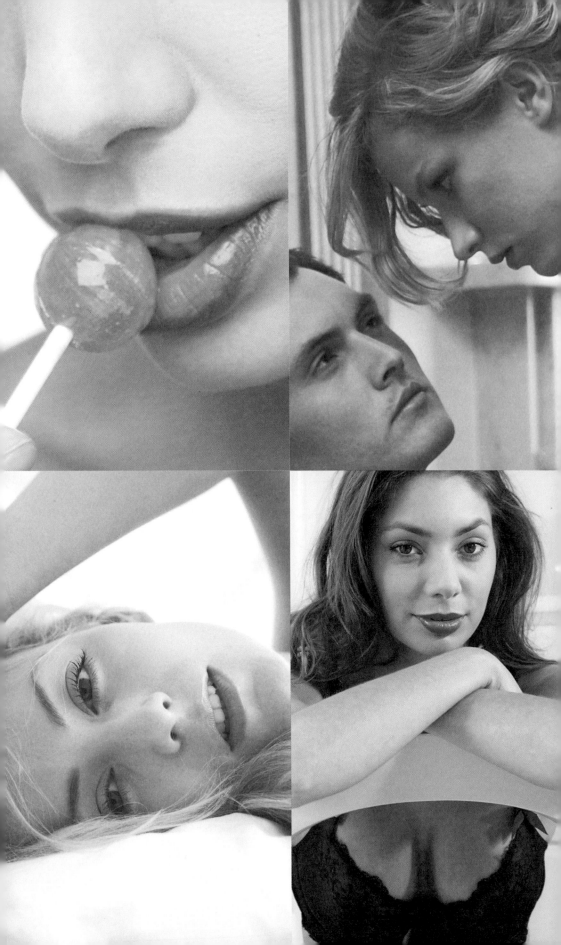

SECRETS OF ...
Flirting

+ **MAKE IT PUBLIC** Flirt outrageously with your man in front of his friends. I've found that my lover adores the flattery when his friends can see I've only got eyes for him.

+ **LOOK HIM IN THE EYE** ... and hold his gaze. Don't speak. Even if you know each other inside out, prolonged eye contact feels unsettling and exciting. Gaze appreciatively at his lips, too (I always imagine giving my lover a hot, sexy kiss at this point). Now look into his eyes again – let him see your desire.

+ **BE NAUGHTY** Use symbolic gestures: purse your lips around a straw as you're drinking or suck a lollipop and gaze up at him as you do so. Briefly lick your lips or twine your hair in your fingers.

+ **USE MIRRORING** If he takes a sip of his drink, take one, too. If he changes position, change yours to match. Unconsciously, he'll be flattered that you're so highly in tune with him. In my experience, it's good to keep your moves subtle. Go for reflection rather than obvious mimicry of his gestures and body language.

+ **LAVISH HIM WITH COMPLIMENTS** Look your partner in the eye and tell him how funny, intelligent, sexy or loveable he is. Most importantly, make sure you mean it.

+ **TEASE HIM** Try playfully withholding sex. It'll make him feel he's got to seduce, entice and woo you. When he suggests going to bed, be cheeky and ask him exactly what he's offering before you agree. I try to never be a sure thing (even if I am!).

SEX ON THE MIND

Want a way to become instantly sexier? Start thinking about sex more. I've discovered the more naughty thoughts I have, the more sexual attention I get from my lover, partly because I initiate sex more, and partly because I'm already raring to go when he's in the mood. I also find I start giving out more sexy vibes to men in general (which is fantastic for some innocent flirting).

THINK SEXY

Make sex your new hobby: think about it, plan it, read about it. Try any or all of the following:

+ Plan a "sex date" with your lover – then lose yourself in erotic anticipation before the event. Imagine the things you'll do; your seduction techniques and the positions you'll try. Put fresh sheets on the bed, arrange some candles on the bedside table and fill the room with fragrant flowers or spray perfume on the bed linen.

+ When you have an idle moment, think a few sexy thoughts. Reminisce about a favourite erotic encounter or dream up a sexual fantasy. I often revisit a holiday I had in Greece (one steamy night on a rooftop, in particular). Share your thoughts with your lover by text, email or letter. My lover always enjoys getting texts that begin: "Hey, do you remember that time we …"

+ Keep some erotic reading beside the bed – hidden away in a drawer if you prefer. Be naughty: go to bed and read it in the middle of the day. If you feel inspired, write your own erotic story or poem.

+ Make sex a conversation piece with female friends – ask if they've ever tried a particular sex position/sex toy/oral sex technique.

SENSUALIZE YOUR LIFE

When I start thinking sexy, I become more sensual. I wear perfume to bed, give my lover sensual massages and make food to share in bed – feeding each other chocolate cake and cream is a favourite.

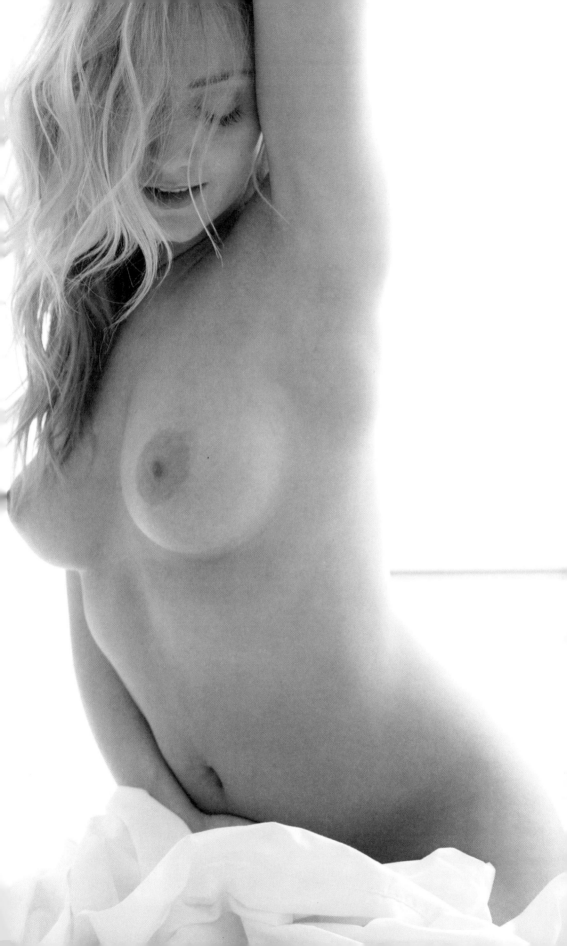

SECRET CONFESSIONS

Outdoor seduction ...

Shortly after we first started going out, my lover took me on a very sexy picnic in the countryside. Instead of sandwiches, he packed cream, honey, strawberries and champagne. I knew things were going to become fun when he started drizzling the honey on me. But for me, the highlight was just being naked outdoors with the sun on my body and the grass tickling my skin. I've always found something very sexy about being close to nature. As I went on to discover, I'm not alone:

"I went on a walking holiday with my boyfriend and we found ourselves on a remote beach sheltered by a high cliff. There was no-one around for miles and my boyfriend, who's a keen photographer, suggested that I strip off so he could take pictures of me. I found it so sensual to lie naked in the sand or pose on rocks. Both of us got incredibly turned on and ended up having wild sex in the sea."

"Forests do it for me. I love the idea of sneaking off into the woods for secret sex, which I used to do with my first boyfriend. I don't know whether it's the possibility of getting lost, being discovered or the naughtiness of being taken up against a tree. I find it very exciting."

"We climbed a mountain once on holiday. We were so exhilarated by getting to the top, we made love standing behind a rock. The lack of comfort didn't matter – it was one of the best sexual highs (!) I've ever had. Sex with a view is amazing."

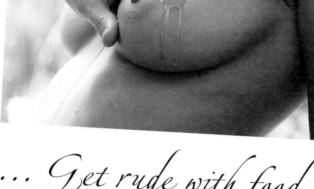

... Get rude with food

HIS TURN-ONS

To seduce your lover you need to know what turns him on. There are lots of myths about male sexuality, but the truth about male turn-ons is often surprising. I've found that rather than fantasizing about the perfect woman, men are far more likely to want to have a fun, sexy time in bed with someone they care about.

LOVE YOUR BODY AND GET NAKED

So you don't have the body and looks of a supermodel? It doesn't matter. Lots of male friends and lovers have told me that the best libido-starter is a fit, healthy body that a woman shows off with pride – and having a relaxed attitude and a body weight that feels and looks right is a lot sexier than being skinny or diet-obsessed.

Feeling comfortable with your shape and size is crucial if you are to have relaxed and pleasurable sex. One close male friend told me that one of the biggest turn-offs in bed for men is a woman who's constantly trying to conceal the bits of her body she's ashamed of – instead of going with the flow of sex, she's avoiding a certain sex position because she doesn't want to reveal her bum or belly.

The simple truth is that men love the sight and feel of a naked woman (try stripping for him; see pages 28–31). Plus they love a woman who's uninhibited enough to "go for it" and really enjoy sex. Hurrying to hide under the covers won't encourage him to ravish you. Joyously offering him your body – however imperfect – will.

SECRET TIP: *Men love the messy and wild look, so forget about your hair and make-up. Let yourself get dishevelled in bed. Tousled hair and flushed cheeks are hot.*

MOAN AND GROAN FOR HIM

Over time I've discovered that I don't have to offer my lover a set of perfectly honed sex techniques. Okay, he won't complain if I tirelessly pulsate my tongue on his penis, or deliver hand skills that match his own masturbation techniques. But one of the biggest turn-ons for men is witnessing your pleasure: he'll simply love the sight of your face in a state of erotic bliss as he touches you. So don't rush to impress your lover with your sexual repertoire – sometimes just responding to his lovemaking techniques will be enough.

A big turn-off for men is a woman who doesn't respond at all – so make all the noise you want. An ecstatic moan can go a long way to making him happy. And if he brings you to orgasm (whether it's with his penis, hand or mouth), he'll be as thrilled as you are.

SECRET TIP: *Whenever you have a peak lust moment, meet your lover's gaze and hold it for a few seconds. Sharing pleasure through eye contact is explosively intense.*

DISCOVER WHAT THRILLS HIM

Whether it's thigh-nibbling, hair-pulling or ear-nuzzling, most of us have personal triggers that turn us on and tip us over the edge. If you make the effort to discover your lover's special turn-ons, you'll be able to turn him to putty and pay him the compliment of truly understanding him sexually.

If your lover doesn't yet know his triggers, have fun helping him find them. For visual stimulation, try going to bed wearing erotic lingerie and stilettos, or doing a sexy dance for him; if he's highly sensitive to touch, try exploring every bit of his skin with your finger-tips. Give him treats that appeal to each one of his five senses – you'll quickly discover what makes him moan. If you've found a technique or touch that takes your lover from zero to 60 in seconds, use it sparingly. Don't let sex treats become predictable.

SECRET TIP: *Men like outrageously naughty lingerie, but some also find plain white undies an incredible turn-on – maybe it's the innocent and virginal overtones. Try slipping into bed in a pair of simple white cotton briefs and a vest.*

UNLEASH YOUR EXHIBITIONIST

In my experience men love to be voyeurs. They're naturally stimulated by what they see – so whether you walk around in your panties or do a striptease (see pages 28–31) – you can turn their lust for the visual to your advantage. The challenge for most of us is to find our inner exhibitionist and then make her centre stage.

If you don't count yourself as a natural exhibitionist, and want to develop your "look-at-me" skills, read on ...

MAKE FRIENDS WITH THE MIRROR

Before I put on any kind of show for my lover, I find it helps to get to know myself in the mirror. Rather than just standing face-on, try out a variety of naked poses and moves: raise your hands above your head; turn around and look over your shoulder; or bend over (keep your back in a straight line and your legs apart). Try dancing, too. Even if you feel silly, you'll quickly become comfortable with your own image. You'll also learn to judge what you like doing and what you don't and, importantly for your self-confidence, what looks good.

SECRET TIP: *For a fast and effective way to overcome shyness, try masturbating in front of the mirror.*

BUILD UP SLOWLY

Once you've found your confidence in front of the mirror, start working exhibitionism into everyday life:

• Wander round the house wearing something provocative. Try a thigh-skimming dress and no underwear, or whatever makes you feel confident and sexy.

• Make a point of undressing in front of your partner when you're getting ready for bed – relish the feeling of his eyes upon you.

- Inject sexiness into the way you sit, stand and walk. Visualize a woman you consider sexy and copy her moves.
- Straddle your partner's lap when he's not expecting it.
- Try sexual positions that put the spotlight on you, such as the cowgirl position – he lies flat on his back and you hop astride. Bask in the attention.

SECRET TIP: *It's not just women who like seeing their lovers in uniform. Try dressing up in a sexy costume with a "power" theme: policewoman, combat girl or girl gangster.*

DEVELOP AN ALTER EGO

Sometimes it's easier to be an exhibitionist if you have an alter ego: quiet office worker by day, sex kitten by night. Props and clothes can help you get into character. Try picturing the kind of person you want to be (for example, vamp, harlot, feminine goddess), then dress the part. Imagine that you can literally step into someone else's shoes. As a friend of mine once confessed: "I just have to put on my heels, black basque, stockings and a cat mask and I can crawl across the floor with no inhibitions." But bear in mind that, although costumes can help, they're not essential. Ultimately, it's a new attitude and persona you're trying to cultivate, rather than a new wardrobe.

SECRET TIP: *Men associate naughtiness with redheads and blondes. If you're a brunette, it might be liberating to wear a wig occasionally!*

LEARN TO SHOW OFF

Now that you've developed your exhibitionist streak, there are plenty of ways you can use it to seduce your partner. Try dancing or stripping for him. Or if you're in an adventurous mood, try lap dancing or chair dancing (see the routine on pages 30–31). You can also be an exhibitionist without even being in the same room as your lover by talking dirty on the phone (see page 32).

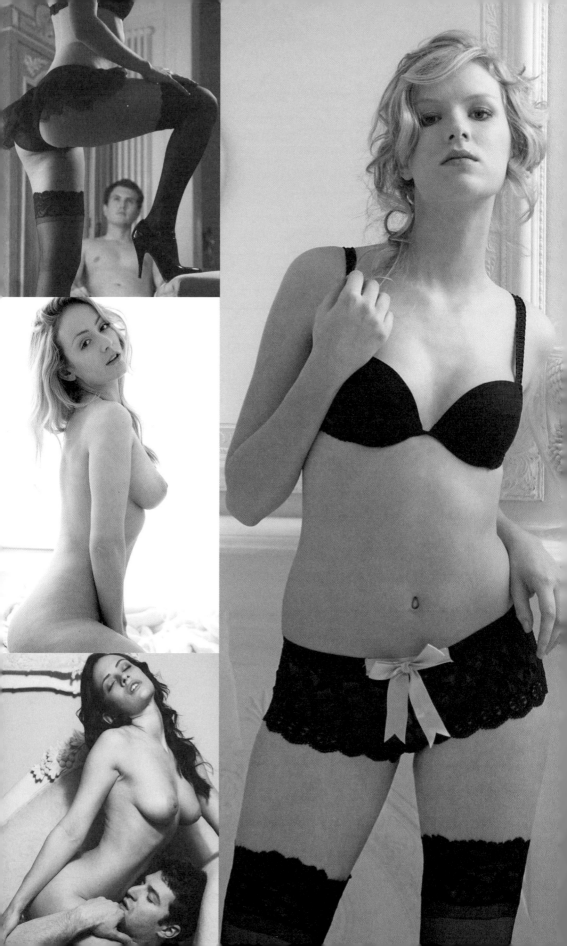

SECRETS OF ...

Sexual confidence

+ **KNOW YOUR SEXUAL SELF** Know what makes you climax (and what doesn't), know where your G-spot is (see page 56), know what turns you on. Don't wait for your lover to unlock your sexuality – make sure you get there first.

+ **USE THE POWER OF YOUR IMAGINATION** Close your eyes and picture yourself as a sexy goddess – someone who's comfortable in her own skin; who adores giving and receiving pleasure; and who loves to touch, tease, flirt and dance. Be that person in bed tonight.

+ **DISCOVER YOUR "HOT TIMES"** Lots of women have told me that they feel sexy around mid-cycle (when they ovulate). I've noticed it, too. Keep a diary of your cycle, and then tie in a date with your lover.

+ **COMPLIMENT YOURSELF** Look in the mirror and say "I've got great breasts." "I'm gorgeous." "I love my hair." "My curves are sexy." Keep a "mental bank" of the compliments people pay you.

+ **SHOW OFF YOUR SEXINESS** Dress to show off your assets; connect with people through eye contact; be tactile; laugh and smile; try to be uninhibited and proud of your body when you're naked.

+ **TREAT YOURSELF** ... to a sex toy, a slinky dress, a pampering session or lovely lingerie (wear it even when no-one will see it).

+ **STOP WISHING, START ACTING** Wish you were slimmer/ younger/prettier? Make a list of the things you'd do (both in bed and out) if you could attain your ideal appearance. Now do them anyway.

SEXY STRIPPING

If you want to wield sexual power and send him cross-eyed with lust, there are few better erotic treats than a striptease. And if, like me, you don't have a perfect body, don't worry: your lover will be so busy delighting in the show, he won't be casting a critical eye over you.

PRACTICE MAKES PERFECT

Your striptease will benefit from a dress rehearsal. I've made some comical mistakes in the past (all part of the fun), so learn from me. For example, don't wrestle with tops that need to be pulled over your head; wear garments that can be sexily unzipped or unbuttoned. And, rather than trousers (difficult to step out of with dignity), wear a skirt or dress that can be shimmied down your body. Stockings are a must, as they can be smoothed slowly down your thighs. Remember the mirror is your best friend – it'll teach you how to be stunning. To get started, steal some tricks from stripping scenes on the internet. Or turn to Hollywood: watch Demi Moore in *Striptease*, for example. You can also turn the page to see some fabulous stripping poses.

Aside from playing a sexy soundtrack and ensuring the lighting is flattering, you'll need a chair. You can rest your foot on it while you unzip your kinky boots and unroll your stockings, and sit on it Christine Keeler-style (see page 31).

PERFORM FOR HIM

The secret of sexy stripping is attitude rather than moves. You want to project an attitude of self-confident sexiness – revel in your sexual power. Show your lover that you're having fun by holding his gaze; tease him by getting close then moving away; stick your bum out and wiggle it; lean over him so he has a great close-up view of your cleavage. Once the striptease is over, I like to have a surprise for him to discover on my naked body. For example, a temporary tattoo on my thigh or a navel jewel. Don't let the show end there. Undress him, too.

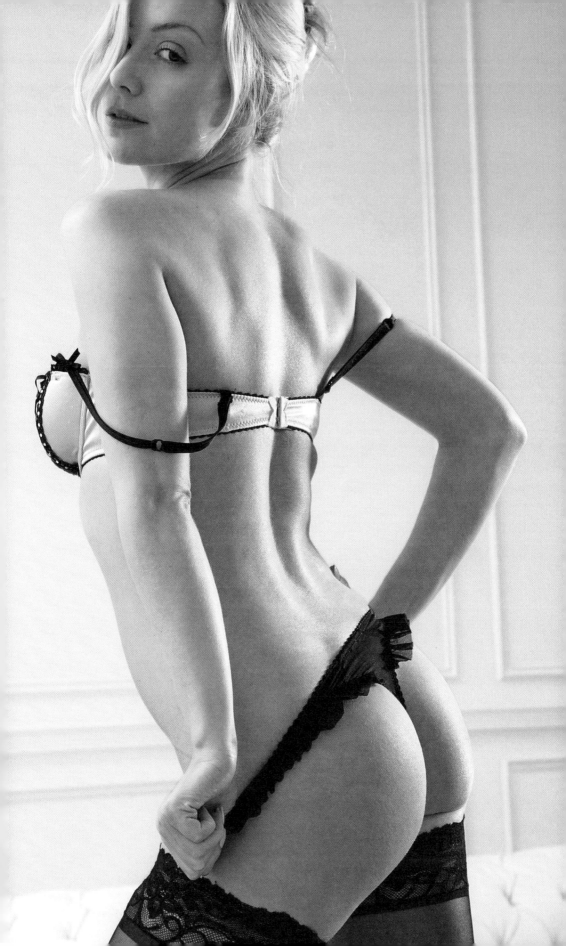

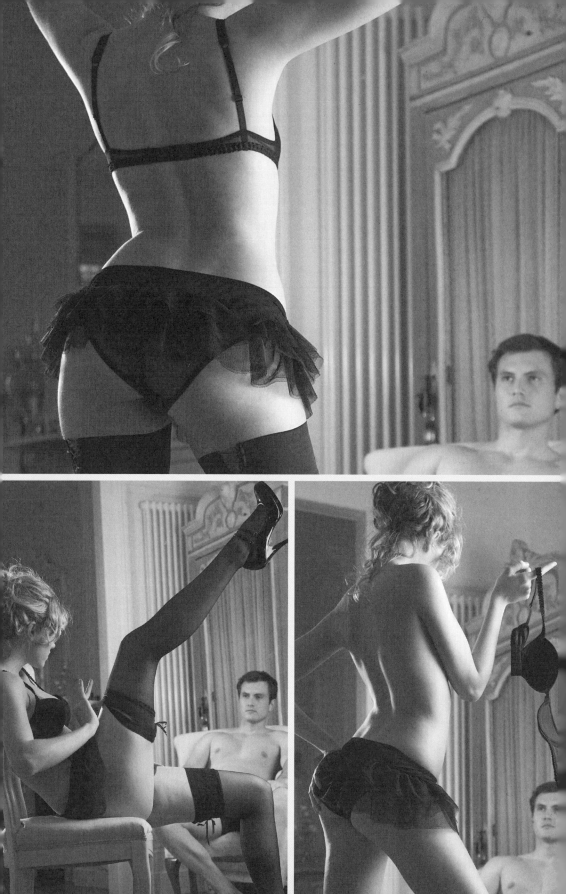

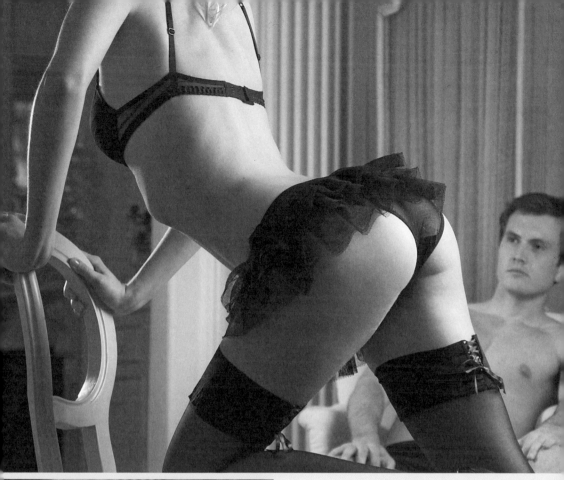

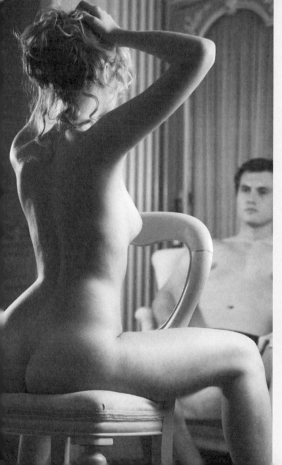

STUNNING STRIPTEASE

BEFORE YOU BEGIN, let yourself be inspired by the classic moves shown here. Make sure your lover is sitting comfortably, switch the music on and begin your performance. Remember: use the chair to show off your body. Lean against the back and stick your bum out, then sit down and raise a leg. Trace the outline of your thighs as you push your stockings off. Tease your lover by making your moves slow and tantalizing. When you take your bra off, dangle it provocatively before dropping it. End your striptease facing him so he can feast his eyes upon you.

TALK DIRTY

My first boyfriend converted me to the joys of talking dirty. We'd gone to bed and I was feeling sleepy, but my tiredness soon vanished as he whispered a few choice words in my ear, followed by "Open your legs, I want to lick you." The sex that followed was really hot.

It surprised me because I hadn't thought of myself as a talk-dirty-in-bed kind of person. But once I experienced the naughty power of words, I suddenly got it: sex felt more adult, X-rated and exciting. Plus I found that:

+ Dirty talk can intensify your orgasms. In fact, if your sex life is feeling jaded, some salacious chat can quickly turn things around.

+ You can change your entire sexual persona instantly. There's no faster way to go from good girl to wicked girl. You don't need exotic outfits, sex toys or kinky whips – just the simple erotic power of your own voice can be transforming.

+ You've got a readily available sex tool at your disposal – any time, any place. Although it might not be legal to have intercourse in a public place, there's no law to stop you whispering expletives to each other. No-one else need know.

+ If your lover's erection is flagging, dirty talk can send blood rushing straight to where it's needed. And if it isn't flagging, your X-rated words will make him feel like he's bursting at the seams and give him a turbo-charged orgasm.

+ If you're apart, you can have amazing telephone sex. Try phoning him late at night. Tell him you're naked, touching yourself and can't stop thinking about him.

+ If you usually have sweet, lovey-dovey sex, dirty talk can charge up your sex life and make you see each other in a completely different – and more exciting – light.

+ Dirty talk can be explosive in the moments leading up to orgasm. Just tell him in your own words that you're about to hit the peak – he'll love hearing about the pleasure he's giving you.

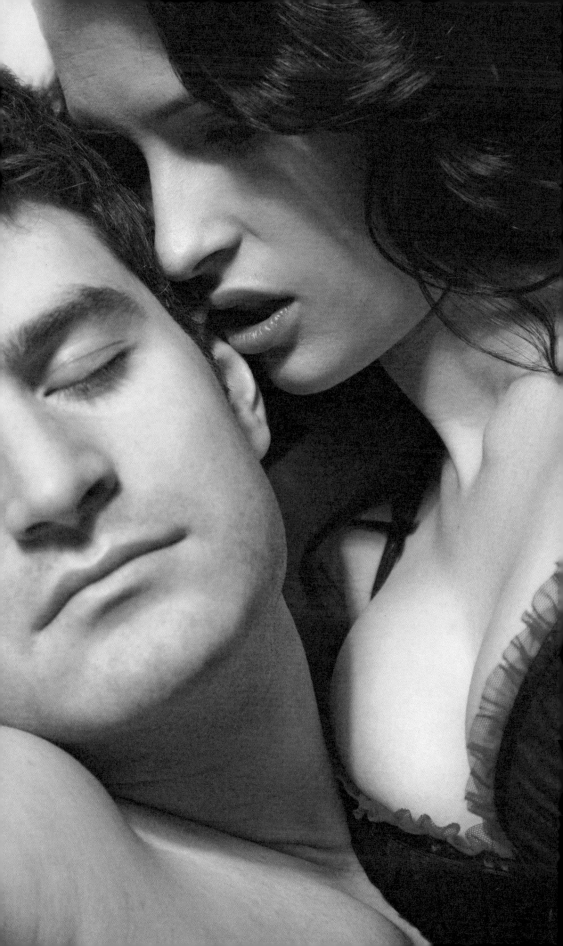

FEELING TONGUE-TIED?

If you're a novice when it comes to talking dirty, you can look forward to the thrill of leaving your comfort zone and pushing back the boundaries. If you've ever moaned your lover's name or shouted an expletive during sex, you're partly on the road to talking dirty already – you just need to take it a step further. If you don't know where to start and are in need of inspiration, try reading erotic literature. Borrow the lines you find erotic, but, remember that, ultimately, the best dirty talk will be your own. It doesn't have to be sophisticated – it's best when it's authentic, and fuelled by lust and arousal.

Learn to let go – embrace rude language in the bedroom. Okay, you wouldn't want your parents, friends or colleagues to hear you, but it's fine to be sleazy when it's just you and your lover. It becomes a delicious secret for the two of you to share. You don't have to do it every time you have sex – just when you're in the mood. And put aside your fears about him finding you cheap. As one close male friend confessed: "I love it when my girlfriend is filthy, especially because I know it's for my ears only. It really turns me on." *SECRET TIP: Discover your "voice" when you're lying on your own in bed and feeling sexy. Don't think about what you're saying – let a stream of consciousness emerge. No one can hear you. You'll quickly discover your natural erotic vocabulary, then you can thrill your lover with it.*

SIMPLE WAYS TO BE MORE EXPRESSIVE

Often it's not how you say it, but what you say. If you're short of ideas, follow this formula ...

First: describe what you want to your lover. As well as being incredibly erotic, it's a handy way to let him know your turn-ons. For example: *"I want you to kiss me, really softly at first, then deeply and passionately. When I'm ready, slip your hand up my skirt and touch me through my panties. I want to feel your fingertips brushing my clitoris."*

Second: describe the sensations you're experiencing as your lover touches and arouses you. As well as giving him a massive amount of encouragement, it also makes whatever you're feeling more intense. *"Mmmm, I can feel you touching me. It feels so good. I'm tingling. I love it when your fingers brush lightly against me. Wow – that's fantastic. Please don't stop."*

Third: say what you're going to do to your lover. *"I'm going to kiss you slowly all the way from your mouth to your thighs. Then, I'm going to take you in my mouth."*

Throughout a lovemaking session, describe to your lover what you're doing, how it feels and what you want to happen next. You don't have to give a continuous commentary – fill in the gaps with moans, "mmmm"s or fast breathing. And don't get too hung up on the words you're going to use – I've noticed the more turned on I get, the more my tongue loosens. Just relax and you'll soon find that the right words come to you.

It's also a good idea to thoroughly know your partner's sexual tastes and attitudes beforehand, and for him to know yours. If there's an area of sex that's contentious, you'll know to avoid it. Then you can relax and relish the naughtiness.

FIND YOUR VOICE

The stereotypical female dirty-talk voice is husky and breathless – if you can do this, fine. If you can't, find something that comes naturally. Let your voice convey your emotion. For example, whisper if you're feeling shy, moan if you're excited, or just talk in your normal voice. The suggestive charge in your voice will develop naturally as things get hotter.

SECRET CONFESSIONS

Phone sex

I was on my way to a dinner date with my lover when he called to say he was running late. He told me to go and sit at the table and order some wine. Rather than hanging up at this point he carried on chatting, telling me in increasingly salacious detail all the wicked things he wanted to do to me. He was still talking when I was at the table sipping wine. For 15 minutes I said "uh huh" and "oh, really?" as the restaurant filled up with prim-looking diners. I could feel a slow blush rising up me. Several times I said "I have to go now", but he wouldn't let me. In fact any sign of embarrassment spurred him on to new heights of depravity. I secretly loved it. It reminded me what a titillating tool the phone is. Here are some confessions from other phone sex fans:

"My boyfriend has a deep, gravelly voice that's perfect for phone sex – it's aroused me since the day we met. It's strange to say, but I almost enjoy phone sex as much as sex in the flesh. I dress in my sexiest underwear, then lie in bed caressing myself while I wait for him to call (we agree a time so we can both get the thrill of anticipation). I love the moment when the phone rings – I still get butterflies. And when I pick up he never bothers with saying hello – he just says my name softly. I've never told him how aroused I get by this."

"My partner and I once decided to phone a sex phone line out of sheer curiosity. It was more funny than erotic – neither of us could take the breathy panting seriously. But it did have an amazingly sexy side-effect, freeing us of our own inhibitions. Now phone sex is a really fast way for both of us to have an orgasm when we're apart. It brings out our filthiest sides."

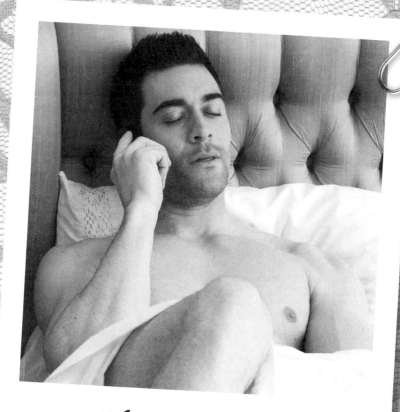

... Thrill him with words

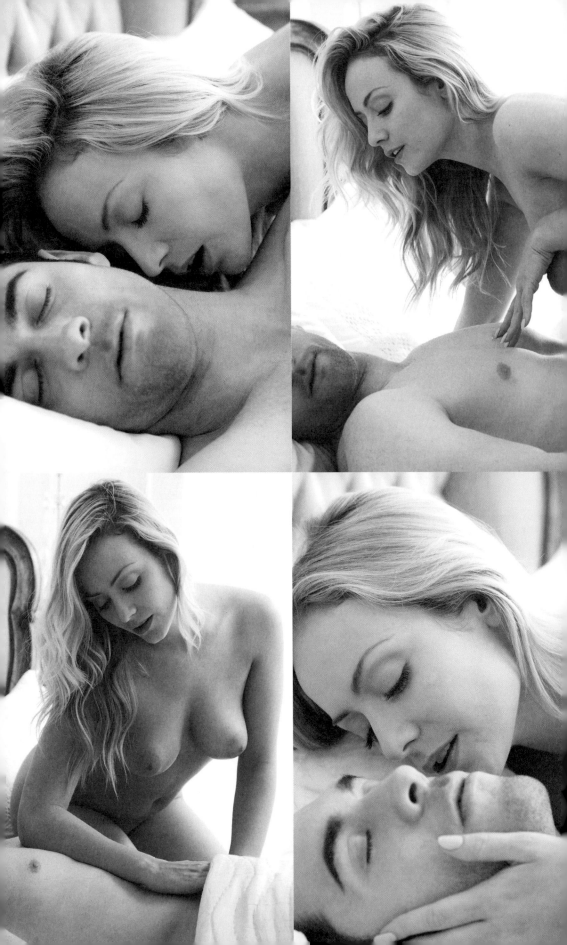

SECRETS OF ...
A hot relationship

+ **PLAY THE COMPLIMENT GAME** You give him a compliment and he returns it – now just keep going. Sex is great when you're both high on intense mutual admiration.

+ **MAKE MORNINGS SEXY** If sex was fantastic last night, whisper in his ear when he wakes up. For example, "I loved what you did to me last night, especially the way you dominated me." Then let your hands drift down to discover his morning erection.

+ **BE PLAYFUL** When you go for dinner with friends, agree a "trigger" word in advance, such as "delicious", "taste", "sauce". When someone says the word, you must caress each other under the table or kiss.

+ **DON'T BE A SLOB!** On a night in, don't just throw on your jogging pants and old T-shirt. Wear something that outlines your breasts, bum and hips, so that he longs to stroke your curves.

+ **DO IT ANYWAY** There will always be times when you're tired and not in the mood – but get passionate anyway. I guarantee that after five minutes of heavy smooching, your body will catch up.

+ **BE SEXY OUTSIDE THE BEDROOM** Let your lover know you think he's hot all the time, in bed and out. Trail your fingers across his bum; caress his chest and belly; nuzzle his neck.

+ **REMEMBER THE FIRST TIME** Describe to him the time you first met/kissed/made love. Tell him in graphic detail all the things you fancied about him – and still do.

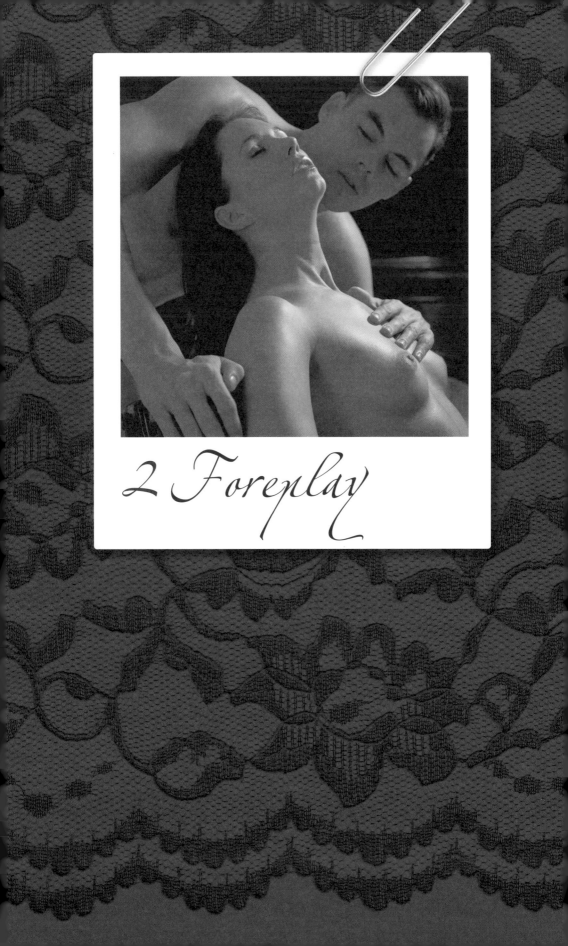

2 Foreplay

THE ART OF AROUSAL

Now you've seduced each other and sex is definitely on the cards, you've got the exciting job of taking each other to a pitch of arousal, through foreplay. Without doubt, my favourite foreplay is kissing – it takes me to another dimension. It should be slow and exploratory at first, then build up to a passionate tongue-twining crescendo. If my lover cups my face or caresses the small of my back, even better.

Whatever your favourite type of foreplay, do it wholeheartedly. Whether you're caressing/fellating/sensually massaging your partner, don't treat it as a means to an end. Do it passionately, as though there's nothing you'd rather be doing in the world. Without rushing, get each other to the point where you both want sex *now*.

GET INTO THE GROOVE

Good foreplay is like good dancing, so find a natural rhythm and don't worry too much about the moves. Forget scripted ideas of what foreplay "should" be. You don't have to do it lying down, for example. For a sense of naughtiness, I like making out while leaning against the bedroom door. And sometimes it's fun to be boisterous and rough as well as gentle and loving.

By the way, there's no rule to say that foreplay has to lead to sex. Sometimes I've found it so exciting, it becomes the main event. Maybe it's the way my lover is caressing my clitoris or the way I'm touching his penis – it's just too good to interrupt. Think of it as a meal – what you thought was just the starter turns out to be so delicious you have it for the main course and dessert too.

My female friends told me their top foreplay moments:
"He sucked my fingers while he caressed me – it drove me crazy."
"He pushed my legs apart and just breathed hotly on my clitoris – it was amazing. Then he started teasing me with little cat licks."
"In the shower – he wrapped his arms around me from behind and started playing with my nipples. Then I turned round and went down on him."

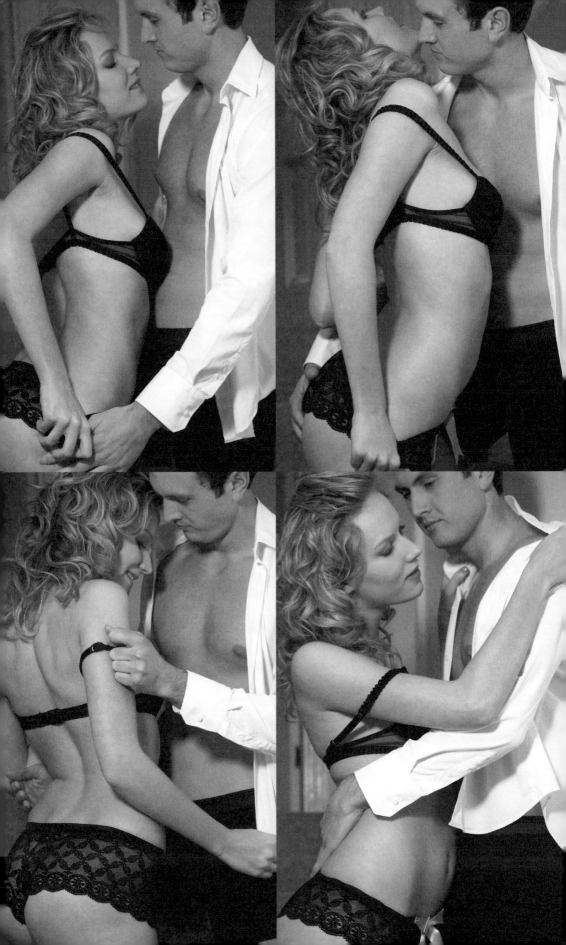

MIND-BLOWING MASSAGE

A sensual full-body massage is the perfect build-up to sex for many men. The sensation of your fingertips caressing, playing and stroking him all over can electrify his senses and open him up to pure pleasure. And when you've finished, he can have the thrill of caressing your naked body in return.

I usually start by lighting some candles in the bedroom (yes, it's a cliché, but it really helps to set the mood and ambience), then I invite him to come and lie down with me. I put a big, pre-warmed towel on the bed for him and – one of my favourite parts – drizzle warm, fragrant massage oil all over his skin. After several minutes of hot and slippery smooching, I push him onto his tummy, sit astride his thighs and start my massage.

SECRET TIP: *I use my breasts to rub the oil in (he finds all that sliding a massive turn on).*

LYING ON HIS FRONT ...

Begin with long, flowing strokes – hands flat – that begin just above his buttocks and go all the way up to his shoulders. Then swirl your hands back down along the sides of his body. Keep doing this and don't break contact even for a second (it disrupts the sensual mood). Imagine you're bringing your lover's skin alive with each stroke.

Now pay attention to his upper back and shoulders – run your fingertips gently over his muscles trying to intuit where he most wants to be touched. Listen out for any pleasurable moans. Gently pull and squeeze the flesh on the top of each shoulder between your fingertips. If there's a tension spot, use your thumbs to smooth, press and apply firm circular pressure. But don't make it your mission to unknot his back – keep the massage sensual and erotic.

Wriggle down his thighs a bit and place a flat palm squarely on each buttock. Now slowly lean forward so that your body weight very gradually transfers itself into your hands. Now slowly lean back.

Repeat this sensational move as many times as you like. Follow up with some deep twisting massage strokes in the centre of his buttocks; either with the flat part of your fist or the heels of your hands.

Now you've opened up sensation in his buttocks, make him glow with eroticism: straddle him on all fours and lower your breasts so they're touching the backs of his thighs. Now glide over his buttocks and up his back. Repeat!

SECRET TIP : *Make sure that you enjoy the massage as much as he does: take little breaks to concentrate on your own pleasure. While he's lying on his front, sit up and stroke your nipples and clitoris. He'll be titillated by the moans of pleasure going on behind his back.*

LOVING HIS LEGS

Let your partner stay on his front while you make his legs tingle with pleasure. Make a "V"-shape between your fingers and thumb, and cruise your hands up his calves and thighs (reduce the pressure as you glide over his knee joints). Enjoy squeezing the powerful muscles of his thighs as your hands slowly pass over them. Keep doing this for as long as you want to, then slowly, imperceptibly, start making your touch lighter. Then switch your stroke so you're dragging the backs of your fingers along your partner's legs. Go all the way up to his buttocks. The beauty of this stroke lies in its ability to sensitize and arouse. Expect to hear lots of "mmms" and "ahhhhs" of pleasure.

And now the feet, which are a massive source of pleasure, second only to the genitals in some men. Tenderly place your partner's foot on your thigh and press all over the sole with your thumbs. You can use your thumbs in several different ways: apply on-the-spot circles; give static pressure on a single point; and sweep or "wipe" along the sole in a smooth line. All of these can have a deeply releasing effect on him and can pave the way for amazingly sensual sex later on. I like to end the foot massage on an especially naughty note: I press his foot

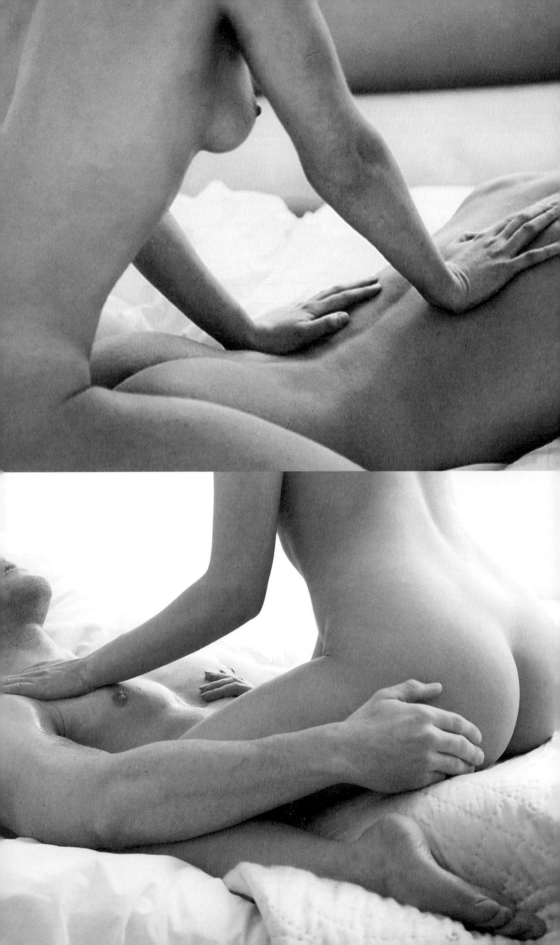

between my legs and make him wiggle his toes against my clitoris. My lover also finds it incredibly erotic to feel my hair tickling his toes. One other sensual technique that will feel great for him: if you have long hair, try twining it tightly around each of your lover's toes to give him a completely novel sensation.

LYING ON HIS BACK ...

Lean down and whisper: "Roll over – I want to touch your front." Check his chest is still slippery with oil and if not, apply more – again, use your breasts to do this if you want to give him a real thrill. Once he's oiled, stroke him with flat palms from the middle of his chest and around the sides of his ribs. Make him melt with the sensuality of your flowing continuous circles.

Gradually extend your circles until they reach as far as his abdomen. Tease him by letting your fingertips stray close to his genitals but never quite touching them. Then brush his penis occasionally, as if by accident.

Once he's relaxed and sensitized, he's extremely likely to get an erection. Give him plenty of encouragement by getting more generous and deliberate with your strokes: smooth your oiled palm along the length of his penis in the direction of his head. Draw swirly shapes on his abdomen before returning to his penis. Include occasional strokes of his perineum, the area just behind his balls. Or lean forward and softly kiss the tip of his penis. In time, let him know how aroused you are too: lean forward to kiss his lips, or moan and writhe. Straddle him and let your genitals brush against his – now's the time to start indulging yourself. Sex will soon be irresistible for both of you.

For a special treat, try a "three-handed massage" in which you slide onto your lover's penis as you massage the front of his body. You simply move on and off him in time with your massage strokes (your vagina acts as the third "hand").

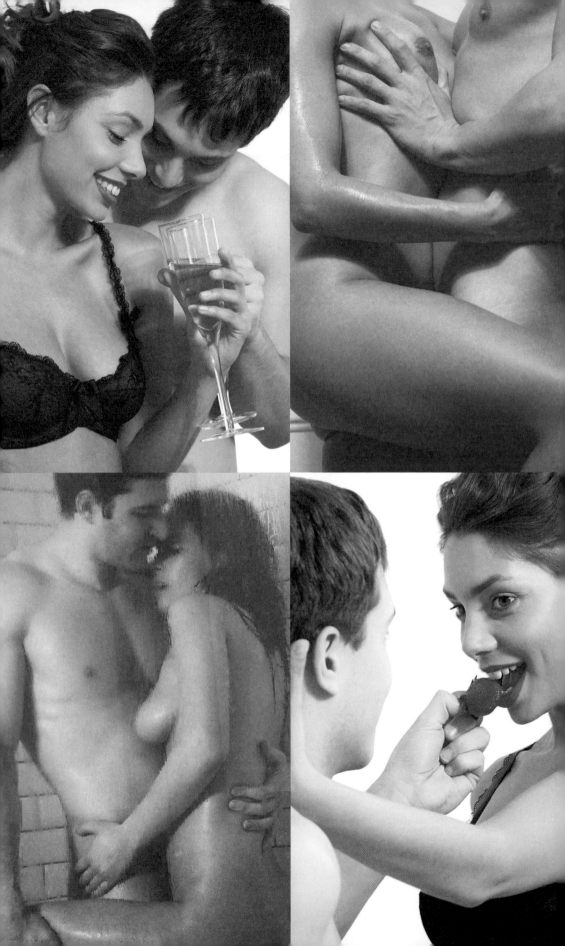

SECRETS OF ...
Aphrodisiacs

♦ **SIP CHAMPAGNE** Alcohol has been called a "false aphrodisiac", because too much can hamper sexual response. My advice is treat it as a romantic luxury and drink it in moderation. Great things have happened when I've begun the evening with a glass of champagne.

♦ **TAKE HIM TO AN OYSTER BAR** Casanova is said to have eaten 50 oysters for breakfast daily. Oysters aside, any food that has an erotic look helps put you in the mood for passion. I love figs, pomegranates, peaches and cherries for their voluptuous naughtiness. Nibbling fruit/licking juice from my lover's naked body is super-sexy.

♦ **GO HERBAL** Many herbs are touted as aphrodisiacs but few actually make the grade. One exception is rhodiola. It's said to not only enhance libido, but to improve physical performance, boost energy levels and combat fatigue – perfect for long, lustful nights.

♦ **USE LAVENDER OIL** Smell has a massively potent effect on desire. I still swoon at the smell of a particular aftershave. Strangely, researchers found that the smell of lavender and pumpkin pie are most stimulating to men. Try them!

♦ **SNIFF HIM** Try having no-holds-barred, sweaty sex. Perspiration secreted during sexual arousal contains pheromones that can act as powerful aphrodisiacs. Prepare for a wild night.

♦ **SPICE THINGS UP** Hot and fragrant spices are reputed to inflame the libido. Ginger is said to be "the food world's Viagra." Pepper, cardamom and chillies are also said to boost sexual desire.

SHARE YOUR FANTASIES

Do you tend to keep your fantasy life tightly under wraps? If so, you could open yourself up to a whole new wonderful world of erotic creativity – just by getting in touch with your sexy thoughts and sharing them with your lover.

I've always found that sex has improved with fantasizing. A really sexy fantasy boosts my libido, gives me more intense orgasms, and makes me feel more adventurous with my lover. And if I confess to something I'm embarrassed about (I once had a thing about firemen), and he goes along with it, I fall in love with him all over again.

If your sex life has been pretty restrained up until now, there's nothing wrong with borrowing or stealing other people's fantasies to get your creative (and other) juices flowing. I always turn to the author Nancy Friday – she's published a huge range of sexual fantasies from the everyday to the downright kinky.

Alternatively, go online with your lover in search of eroticism. And when you find what truly turns you on, don't be ashamed of ravishing your lover and capitalizing on it.

EROTIC REVELATIONS

Having explored the fantasies of others, try sharing your own sauciest wishes (think threesomes/sex in public/domination/dressing up). Discuss how you can bring your fantasies to life or, if that's going too far, find some erotica that enacts your fantasy for you. Read the following confessions friends have shared with me, then add your own.

"I'd love to have an orgasm when I'm out with my boyfriend. I imagine him touching me under the table at a restaurant."

"I fantasize about my boyfriend filming me while I'm masturbating."

"I've often imagined kissing another woman. No one in particular – just a woman who exists in my fantasies."

"Red silk sheets, candles, rose petals, log fire and music as we make love."

"I'd like my boyfriend to blindfold me and then be the boss."

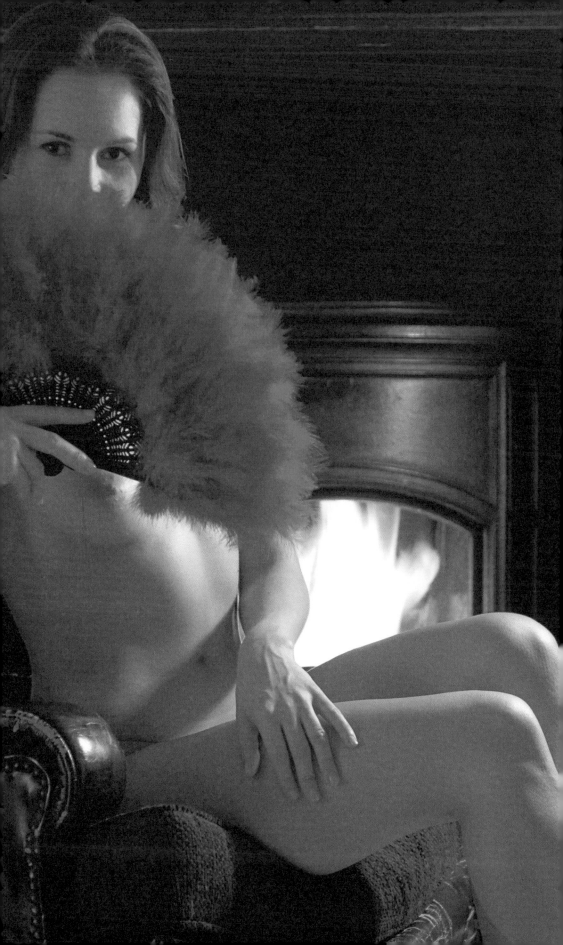

ASK FOR WHAT YOU WANT

I've had the most pleasure in bed when I've asked for what I want. It's incredibly titillating for my lover; and he's usually glad to get some guidance from me. After all, a nice specific request means that he doesn't have the burden of responsibility and guesswork. Despite an air of confidence, men don't always know what women need sexually, especially in my case when it can change from one night to the next.

But most importantly, asking for what you want means you get the right stimulation exactly where, when and how you need it. Which means you'll be incredibly turned on and ready to go – the perfect recipe for raunchy sex.

KNOW WHAT THRILLS YOU

In order to create your erotic wish list, you need to know which buttons/zones you'd like your lover to press/caress. If prioritizing your sexual needs isn't something you're used to, take some time out for private study. Read pages 18–19, Sex on the Mind, to discover the art of self-seduction.

Alternatively, let yourself be inspired by my pick 'n' mix foreplay list: steamy tongue swirls on your clitoris; a long and sensual head and shoulder massage; his hand creeping under your skirt to touch your thigh while he's driving; mutual masturbation; kisses on the tips of your fingers; lovebites; toe-nibbling; breast massage; nipple tweaking; light bondage; passionate kissing.

Don't cheat by asking your partner to do things he'll find easy or that put his pleasure first. Take a deep breath and ask for what you really want – even if it's kinky. If you don't want to look him in the eye and share your wishes, just whisper your desires into his ear during foreplay or while you're having sex. Or try this …

SECRET TIP: *If you discover a technique in this book you want your lover to try, pop a Post-It saying "Tonight?" on the relevant page. Then leave it on his pillow.*

KNOW WHAT TO SAY ...

Drench your requests with praise, encouragement and compliments. Men will thrive on it. For
example, if he hears that you absolutely love a particular sexual technique – and you just want more
of it, or you just want it softer or harder, he'll be
delighted. Criticism is a no-no in the bedroom – it's
a massive passion killer and can result in less sex rather
than better sex.

So try this next time you want to ask something: surround
your request with authentic compliments, look at your lover
mischievously and say: "You're brilliant with your hands – and
there's this technique I'd really like to try ..." or "You did something
amazing with your tongue when you kissed me – I can't stop wonder-
ing how it would feel if you did that to my clitoris."

SECRET TIP: *Men respond well to specifics, so make your requests
as precise as possible. Instead of asking him to "caress you with his
hands and mouth", use words that leave him with no uncertainty.
For example, "I'd like you to put your fingers inside me while you
give me oral sex."*

GIVE HIM A DEMO

I've found that showing my lover what I want speaks a thousand words.
Give him a sexy guided tour of your body or touch yourself in front of
him. Show him your ideal cunnilingus tongue moves by treating the
tip of his finger like a clitoris – swirl, flick or lap your tongue against it
in exactly the speed and rhythm you want. Then offer him a finger or
toe in return so he can demonstrate the perfect fellatio moves.

SECRET TIP: *If a demo feels strange, you can make it into a sexy
roleplaying game. Pretend you're virgins and have to rely solely on
each other to learn about the opposite sex.*

SECRET CONFESSIONS

Erotic witness

I love stories in which people find themselves witnessing an erotic act – and getting helplessly turned on by it. These are two of my favourites:

"My partner and I saw something really erotic at a festival. We were sitting by our camp fire when we saw a couple go into their nearby tent and switch on a torch. The torchlight had the amazing effect not just of illuminating the tent but of creating big theatrical silhouettes of the couple's bodies. As they started undressing we looked discreetly away. But we couldn't resist looking back. The couple were sitting up kissing and stroking. It was like watching an erotic shadow play – we couldn't tear ourselves away. My partner snuggled up behind me and started to kiss my neck and caress my breasts. It was delicious. I'm ashamed to say that we spied on the couple all the way through to their climax scene. Then we had sex ourselves. It was wickedly exciting."

"As a film-maker I was once asked to document a Tantric sex workshop. I went along with a professional mindset – my job was to be the impartial observer and film what was in front of me. In practice, it wasn't so easy. The participants started off fairly tamely with a massage and some sensual dancing. But by the end of the workshop I found myself filming eight naked people all writhing on the floor in erotic abandon. All I wanted to do was drop my camera and join in. I never imagined I'd be so aroused by watching others. I'm proud to say I maintained my professional front. But afterwards I rushed home, full of sexual tension, and pounced on my lover."

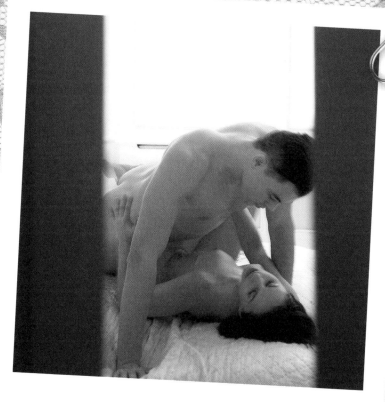

... *Secret voyeur*

HIDDEN HOTSPOTS

For explosive foreplay, find your lover's hotspots – and guide him to yours. Try bypassing the obvious erogenous zones and discover each other's secret ones. I'll start with a classic. Most of us have heard of it, but many women still find it elusive.

IN SEARCH OF THE G-SPOT

The G-spot is best explored when you're extremely aroused – it swells when you're turned on and becomes easier to find. Smooth your lubricated fingertips along the front (belly-side) wall of your vagina until you touch an area that feels like a raised button and is roughly oval in shape. Don't worry if you can't find this – some women experience the G-spot as an area of general erotic sensitivity rather than as a readily identifiable button. Press and massage the G-spot area and see what sensations you experience.

The first time a lover touched my G-spot I was sure I was going to pee – I later discovered this is completely natural. It happens because the G-spot is very close to the urethra. Go with the feelings and see what happens (feelings could range from nothing or mild pleasure all the way through to intense pleasure, vaginal orgasm and female ejaculation). Ask your lover to press and caress your G-spot while you stroke your clitoris. Now relax completely – if you're going to ejaculate, relaxation will increase your chances (see page 111).

AROUSING THE A-SPOT

I needed my lover's help to find this one, because it's high up on the front wall of the vagina. Repeated stroking of the A-spot feels fantastic and increases your chance of vaginal orgasm. Ask your lover to slide his finger/s up as high as he can, feeling for an area that lies by or beyond the cervix. Give him instructions such as "up a bit" or "right a bit" until you feel an area of greater sensitivity, and, as with G-spot stimulation, make sure you're fully aroused before you begin.

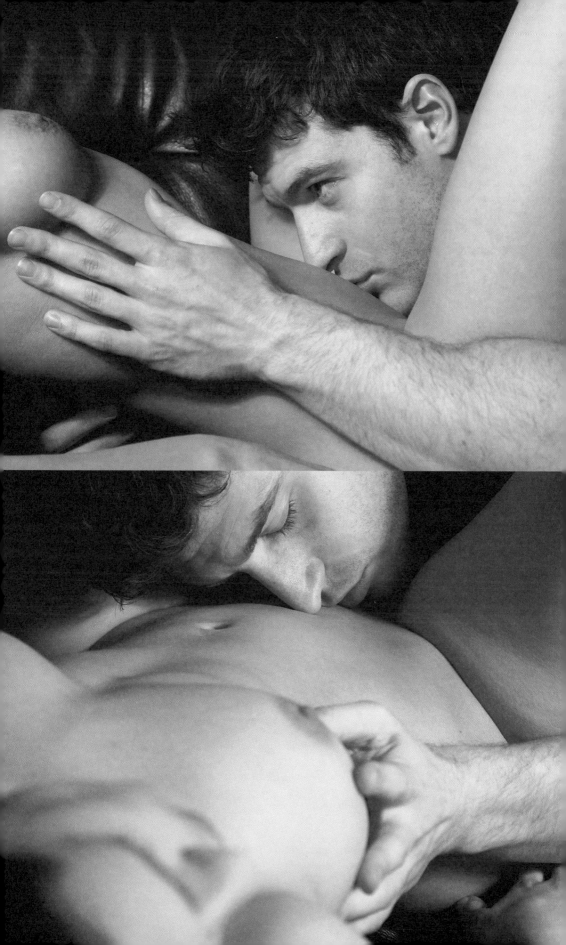

Treat yourself to a G-spotter – this is a vibrator or dildo with a specially curved tip that stimulates the front wall of the vagina. It's designed to target the G-spot, but it works on the A-spot, too.

THE CUL-DE-SAC

While your lover is exploring your A-spot, ask him to take a short detour from the front wall of your vagina to the back – right at the top beyond your cervix. This is the cul-de-sac, and although it doesn't sound very erotic, it's rich in nerve endings and can yield immense pleasure in some women. It's vital to be fully turned on before you start exploring – for comfort and because the cul-de-sac only becomes accessible during peak arousal.

Ask your partner to slide his fingers up as far as he can along the back wall and tell him when he touches an area that makes you gasp. Then simply lie back and enjoy while he strokes and caresses this zone. *SECRET TIP: I've found that lying on my back with a pile of pillows under my bum creates the best access for my lover. Sitting right on the edge of the bed and leaning back works, too.*

UNCOVERING THE U-SPOT

The U-spot is easy to find – it's the place where you pee from – and, because both men and women have one, you can take turns to stimulate each other. Try gently circling your finger on each other's U-spots – exactly where the urethra meets the outside of the body, which means just below your clitoris or on the tip of his penis. Use plenty of lubricant so things feel smooth and sensual; and vary the pressure to discover what feels best. Try using the tip of your tongue on each other, too.

SECRET TIP: Cover your clitoris with your hand while he stimulates your U-spot. If his tongue or fingers can't stray there, you'll know that any erotic sensations are coming directly from your U-spot.

PLEASURING THE P-SPOT

The P-spot is the male G-spot. The "P" stands for "prostate", a small organ that encircles the bladder in men – it gets bigger and firmer the closer he gets to ejaculating, and stimulating it is a great way to give him a powerful orgasm.

You can access the P-spot in one of two ways. Either press upwards on his perineum (towards the back; roughly where the vaginal entrance would be in a woman). Or, the more intimate option, slide a finger or two into his rectum and press your fingers toward his belly. Search for an area that feels different from the surrounding tissue (usually around 5–8cm/2–3in up). If you're not sure whether you're touching the correct place, ask your lover how it feels.

Whichever route you take to access the P-spot, massage it using firm static pressure or pulsating pressure. Or try rubbing it. Ask him what he likes best – or just take your cues from his body language and moans. Oh yes – and make your hands slippery with lube. Dry scratchy friction is a turn off. (And my lover also tends to be much more relaxed if I've got short nails!)

SECRET TIP: *P-spot stimulation works best when I multi-task by using my free hand to caress my lover's penis. Or, for the most heady combination, try fellating him, too.*

FINDING THE F-SPOT

You can find his F-spot or frenulum on the underside of his penis when his foreskin is rolled back. It's the super-sensitive band of tissue that joins the foreskin to the glans. Single out this area for special attention during manual and oral sex: use your lips and tongue to push his foreskin back, then flick the tip of your tongue or swirl your lubricated thumb on his exposed frenulum.

SECRET TIP: *Hold a vibrator against his frenulum – keep it on a low setting, at least at first, so he's not overwhelmed. Move it up and down his shaft, too.*

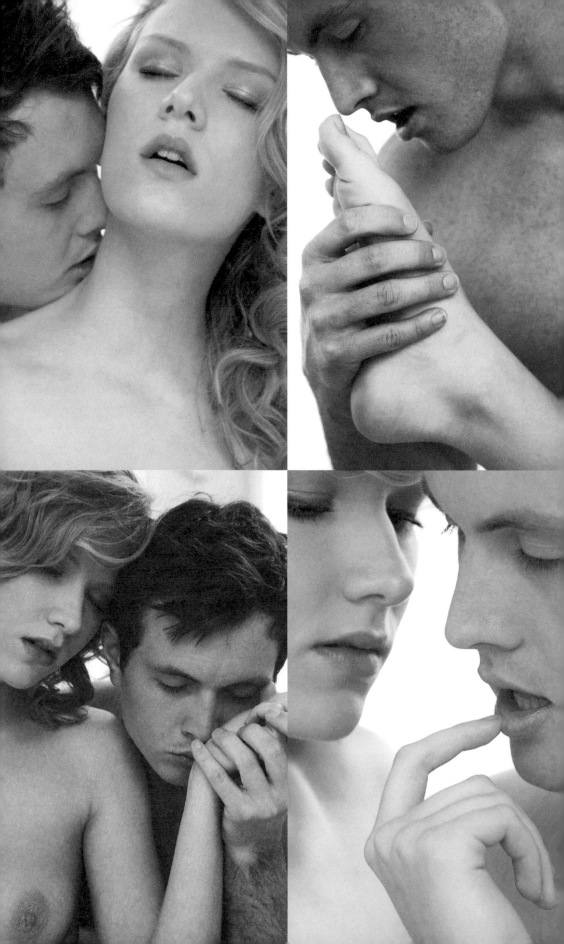

SECRETS OF ...

Erogenous zones

+ **NAUGHTY NECKING** When my lover uses this technique, it always make me swoon with pleasure. He comes up behind me, twists my hair in his hands and lifts it up to expose the nape of my neck. He kisses this amazingly sensual spot, then uses his tongue and teeth to lick, nibble and graze the back of my neck and shoulders. Mmmm ...

+ **WRIST KISS** Ask him to softly press his lips on the inside of your wrist and keep them there. Now get him to pull away and plant a row of really soft kisses along your inner arm.

+ **LIP LOVE** Men tend to concentrate on the clitoris during foreplay, but remind him that your labia are full of nerve endings, too. Ask him to tweak and stroke them for meltingly erotic pleasure.

+ **GIVE EACH OTHER'S TOES A TREAT** Get him to hold your foot firmly and slip his lips over your big toe and slowly slide it in and out of his mouth with plenty of tongue pressure. Now return the favour.

+ **GO DOWN ON HIM** Lie between his legs as if you were giving him oral sex, but, instead, go lower. Nuzzle and kiss the area just behind his balls, his perineum. Inflame him by exploring this neglected area thoroughly with your tongue.

+ **PAY HIM LIP SERVICE** His lips are as sensitive and as greedy for touch as yours. Instead of kissing his lips, gently caress them with your fingers. Run the tip of your index finger around the outline of his lips then slip your finger provocatively into his mouth. Again, he'll associate it with fellatio – a real turn-on.

TANTRA-STYLE PASSION

For sex that's more open, sensual and connected, try the intimate techniques of Tantra. A lot of mystique surrounds Tantric sex but, contrary to what you might expect, the rituals and practices aren't complicated. I've learned lots of simple activities from Tantric workshops – here are some of the most sensual ones.

THE TANTRIC APPROACH

In foreplay terms, Tantra feels like a gift to women – instead of encouraging you to have an orgasm as quickly as possible, you bond slowly with your lover until you reach a blissful peak of physical and emotional intimacy. Even then, you can simply bask in pleasure with no pressure to orgasm. It's said that Tantra "puts the soul back into sex".

You've probably already had Tantric experiences, but you just haven't realized. Think of blissful moments during foreplay or sex when you've felt completely at one with your lover. Rather than thinking about what you're doing, you're just following your body – and tingles of pleasure are running through you. Tantra can give you more moments like these.

One of the things I love about Tantra is that it shows my lover a more feminine way of having sex. He becomes more tender, and I'm more able to lie back and relish the sensations.

CREATE A LOVE NEST

I learnt from Tantra to keep my bedroom clutter-free and more conducive to lovemaking. I make sure there's no dirty laundry, electronic gadgets and other distractions, so that I can relax as soon as I step through the door. I use candles, throws, cushions and exotic-smelling incense, such as cinnamon or sandalwood.

SECRET TIP: One Tantric teacher I know decorates her bedroom with sensual or sexy paintings and photographs. Try taking some sexy shots of your lover, or of the two of you entwined together in a sexy embrace.

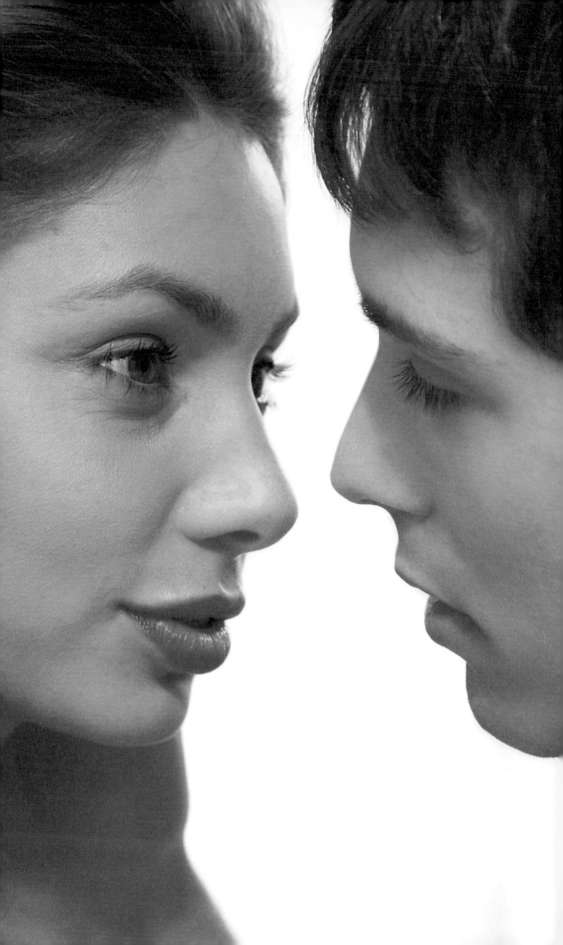

LOSE YOURSELF IN DANCE

Once your love nest is conducive to lovemaking, spend time there relaxing with your lover. Play your favourite music (preferably something rhythmic, trance-like or hypnotic) and, if the mood takes you, get up and dance. You might feel silly (I felt self-conscious at first), but free-form dance is a great way of losing yourself and becoming fully present in your body. So don't worry about impressing your lover with dance moves – the aim is to still your mind through movement. Let your body flow with the music so that it feels as if you're moving without conscious direction from your mind. Think of it like yoga, but without the headstands and backbends.

ENJOY SENSUAL TOUCH

Turn the heating up and the music down and take turns to give each other a slow, sensual massage. Smooth oil into your lover's body with long, loving strokes that flow down the length of his body. Keep your hands in contact with his skin all of the time. Unlike an erotic massage in which you'd aim to build up genital arousal, you're going to include your lover's genitals in the massage, but without singling them out for special attention. Instead, treat his body as though it's one huge erogenous zone.

SECRET TIP: *Make your lover buzz with all-over eroticism by making your touch increasingly light – get to the point where you're barely skimming the skin with your fingertips or fingernails.*

YAB-YUM POSITION

When you're both in a cloud of sensual pleasure, get into the classic Tantric position known as "yab yum" (meaning "position of the mother and father"). If you like this position, you can go on to have sex in it later. Ask your lover to sit cross-legged on the floor, then sit in his lap so that you're facing him with your legs wrapped around his body and your feet behind his back. Once you're in this close Tantric cuddle, hold each other tight and enjoy the sensation of warmth being exchanged between your bodies.

When you're sitting comfortably, start to synchronize your breathing. Inhale and exhale softly through your nose, making your breaths increasingly long, smooth and flowing. When your breath is in a perfect seductive rhythm with your partner's, imagine that any boundaries or obstacles between you are melting away. Let the flow of your combined breath transport you to a place of peaceful love where there's nothing to do, say or think. All you have to do is sit quietly in each other's presence. If you are becoming aroused, embrace the feelings and allow them to intensify, but don't feel that you've got to speed things up, initiate sex or stimulate your partner.

SECRET TIP: *As you become aroused, try gently rocking your pelvis as you sit in your lover's lap.*

SOUL GAZING

As you sit in the yab-yum position, hold each other's gaze. Don't stare each other out – just receive the gaze in relaxed intimacy. Feel any boundaries dissolving – the more you relax, the closer you'll feel. Let your desire build – imagine arousal swirling up from your genitals into your belly. When you're ready, put your hand on your lover's genitals and guide his hand to yours. Caress each other slowly. When and if you have sex, make it close and intimate with small rocking movements that gradually take you higher. Massage each other with your internal muscles (see pages 94–95), and keep gazing.

SECRET TIP: *Try this Tantric kiss: press your lips against his to make a seal. Now blow a soft stream of air into his mouth for him to inhale. Get him to do the same back. Get high on each other's breath.*

SENSATIONAL HANDWORK

Manually stimulating your lover can make you feel like you're up against stiff competition (literally). He'll know first-hand which strokes yield the fastest results. But, remember, fast doesn't always mean best – and this is where you come in. You can offer him the fantastic novelty of a new set of sensations.

SECRET TIP: *One of my close male friends told me that the two most common mistakes women make when handling a penis is using a featherlight touch they can't feel or a vice-like grip that's too intense. To solve this, start with light pressure, then ask your lover if he'd like it tighter. He can then feel free to give you feedback.*

TAKE YOUR POSITION

You may not usually give much consideration to how you're positioned when you stimulate your lover, but it can make a big difference to the sensations he experiences. Plus, I think some positions just feel more erotic than others. Before you start, remember that you may be there for a while, so position yourself to easily swap hands. Try:

+ Sitting between his legs as he reclines on the bed.
+ Kneeling between his legs as he sits in a chair.

Or if you're feeling a bit naughty:

+ Standing behind him and pushing your hand down his trousers.
+ Kneeling over his face or chest with your head pointing in the
  direction of his feet.

DIFFERENT STROKES ...

Make your opening moves teasing. Trail and pitter patter your fingertips over his shaft and testicles as if you're trying to give him goosebumps. As he gets hard, you can take him more firmly in hand with some of the up-and-down strokes that he'd do to himself. You'll need lube (or saliva) from this point to give him delicious, silky sensations – and to create something similar to the warm, slippery touch of your vagina.

When he's got a solid erection, try the "Tunnel of Love": interlock your fingers and wrap your hands around his shaft so he's firmly enclosed in the tunnel of your hands. Position the pads of your thumbs side by side on the underside of his penis and move your hands up and down. Vary the pressure and caress his frenulum (see page 59) with your thumbs as you pass.

To vary things, move on to the "Polishing Stroke": use one hand to grip the base of his penis and the other hand to "polish" his glans. Move your polishing hand in quick, light semi-circles (treat the head of his penis much like you would a lemon if you were trying to juice it; but don't squeeze as hard!).

Mix things up even more with the "Twister". You'll definitely need an extra dab of lube to avoid friction. Make circles with your index finger and thumb on both hands. Now slide these "rings" onto your partner's shaft and twist them in opposite directions. Once you get the hang of it, try twisting and going up and down on his shaft.

If you're going beyond foreplay, ask how he likes to be touched at orgasm – should you pump, squeeze or freeze all motion?

LENDING A HAND IN RETURN

Tell him how much you love his hands on you, too. Most women climax through manual stimulation of the clitoris rather than through the indirect friction of intercourse. For this reason alone, it's important to let him know how valuable his hand skills are. If he's in any doubt about technique, show him how you masturbate, or try "hand-riding" in which he places his hand on top of yours as you stimulate yourself. And if you like G-spot stimulation (see page 56) tell him this, too.

SECRET CONFESSIONS
Mile high

One of my favourite sexual experiences took place on a New York to London flight. My boyfriend fell asleep just after take-off – a fact that alarmed me because I'm terrified of flying. The flight turned out to be really turbulent, and when my boyfriend woke up, I was tired, edgy and anxious. And we were beginning the descent – my least favourite part of the flight. "I've got something for your nerves," he said sleepily. I looked at him doubtfully. He handed me a slim package loosely wrapped in black tissue paper and lace. I slid the lace off and peeked inside – it was a book. On the cover a woman was lying naked with her legs apart and her head thrown back in rapture. The title was something like:"Kinky Stories for Girls."

I thrust the book back in the paper, worried someone would see it. My boyfriend, delighting in my embarrassment, slid it inside a magazine, then opened it at a page he'd bookmarked. He leant close so his lips were nearly touching my ear. "I'm going to read you a story," he whispered in his husky, just-woken-up voice. Then he whispered an incredibly explicit story in my ear. Fittingly, it was about a couple having sex in an aeroplane toilet. As he whispered expletives I could feel my anxiety disappearing and arousal taking its place. When he got to the climactic ending of the story, I was completely turned on. I was desperate for us to be off the aeroplane so that I could kiss and touch him. As we were coming in to land, he got a flimsy aeroplane blanket, pulled it over our laps and leant in to caress me …

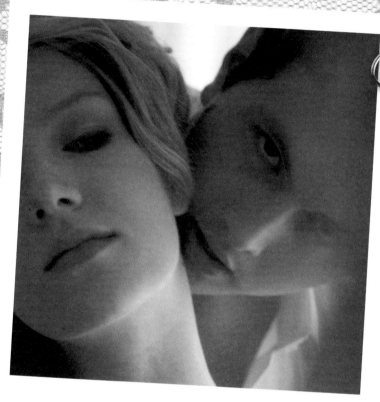

... Sexual adventure

AMAZING ORAL

The ultimate erotic act ... that's how many men think of fellatio. It's hot, wet, tightly targeted stimulation. It's also sublimely intimate – not to mention sexy – when he sees himself encircled by your lips. My lover says that just thinking about a blowjob can give him an erection.

So if you give lots of fellatio, you're likely to have a satisfied, grateful partner on your hands, and one who's willing to be equally generous with you. My favourite secret for giving great oral sex is simple: learn how to enjoy yourself while you're doing it.

GIVE WITH PLEASURE

It's a fact: women don't always relish going down on their lovers. It may be the taste, smell, or the potential for gagging or jaw ache – whatever the issue, there's a way to overcome it.

Sometimes a simple attitude tweak can help. As you head south, think about the tremendous sexual power you're about to wield; the fact that you're about to turn a grown man to putty. See it as an act of love, acceptance and trust. Or take a lesson from Tantric sex in which giving oral sex is seen as a blissful, erotic meditation – a way of immersing yourself in sensation.

If you've got concerns about smell or taste, try these tips: give him a blowjob when he's fresh out of the shower (or while he's still in it); massage him with flavoured lubricant first; or pop a mint in your mouth. If you're worried about gagging or jaw ache, wrap one hand around the base of his shaft so that only the top half of his penis goes in and out – that's the most sensitive bit anyway.

GET AROUSED

You'll give a much better blowjob if you're properly aroused yourself. Make sure you're really turned on, and let one hand linger on your clitoris as you lick him. For the ultimate in reciprocal pleasure, try a 69. Choose the relaxing version in which you both lie on your sides.

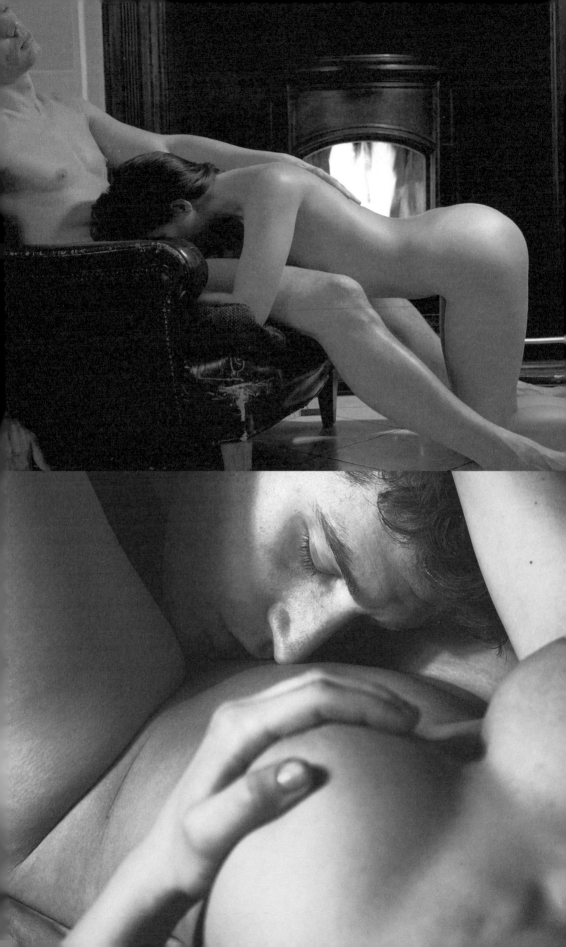

MOUTH STROKES

I find this sexy opener to a blowjob really turns my lover on: kneel in front of him while he's fully dressed and trace the outline of his penis with your fingertips. Then pull his trousers down and press your lips to his genitals through the fabric of his underwear – the heat of your breath and the "near-but-far" feeling will be incredibly enticing for him.

Next, gently coax his penis from his pants and slide it into your mouth. If it's not hard yet, treat this as an advantage – it means you can take the entire length of his shaft in your mouth and seal your lips around the base. This is something that's not easy when he's fully erect. He'll enjoy it because it gives the novel feeling of being completely swallowed up – plus there's the excitement of being able to grow in your mouth.

When he's reached his full potential, you can begin your blowjob in earnest. To give a standard blowjob, seal your lips around your lover's penis, create mild suction with your mouth and tongue and then bob your head up and down (hold him steady with one hand). At the beginning and end of a blowjob, it's good to have a consistent rhythm. But keep him on his toes in the mid-part by varying your moves, speed and pressure.

SECRET TIP: *Drive him crazy with "airbrushing". Hover above his erection and gradually lower your mouth along his shaft without touching him. Caress him with your hot, steamy breath as you descend. Wait until he begs before you enclose him firmly in your mouth. Or be mean and pull away for a detour.*

MAKE IT REALLY SPECIAL

To give an extra-special blowjob caress his testicles, perineum or anus as you go, and vary your mouth moves. Swirl your tongue around his glans on your upward strokes; flick your tongue all over his shaft and testicles; lick him as if you're trying to sculpt an ice-cream; and use your hand and mouth in tandem. Let him see the action,

too (I find that this really ramps up my lover's enjoyment). If you've got long hair, throw it back to give him a clear view. Best of all, look him rapturously in the eyes.

Another extra-special move is irrumatio – the naughtier version of fellatio. Instead of moving your lips up and down on his stationary penis, invite him to thrust in and out of your stationary mouth. Do it with him standing and you kneeling.

THE ULTIMATE SURPRISE

We often pay a lot of attention to fellatio technique, but neglect the art of timing. Men find unexpected blowjobs incredibly exciting. My lover is really turned on when I surprise him with a blowjob in a semi-public place. Whereas penetrative sex can be tricky to execute in public, oral sex can be faster and more discreet. But a risqué venue isn't essential. I once went down on my lover while he was sitting on a chair doing his accounts. It was quite clear which activity he enjoyed most.

DEEP THROAT

Deep throat seems to be one of those sex tricks that sounds amazing but doesn't actually deliver much (at least in my experience). Instead of the classic 70s version, try the cheat's version: just extend the reach of your mouth by adding the well-lubricated tunnel of your hand. Then enclose his penis in your extended "mouth" and "suck" him feverishly.

Or, if you're a stickler for tradition, this is how to do the original: lie back on a bed and dangle your head over the edge (this creates a straight passage between your mouth and throat). He should kneel by the bed and enter your mouth slowly.

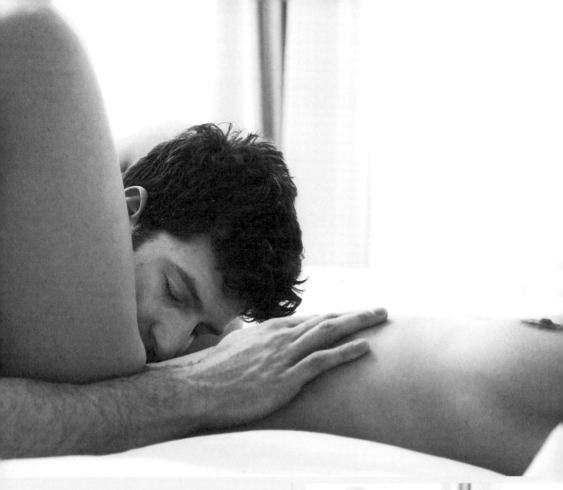

ORAL SEX FOR YOU

LYING ON YOUR BACK with him between your legs has a lot to recommend it. It's really comfortable and relaxing, and the sensations are amazing. But try experimenting with other positions, too. Lying on your tummy while he licks you from behind feels fantastically naughty. And any position in which you're on top gives you the exquisite thrill of domination.

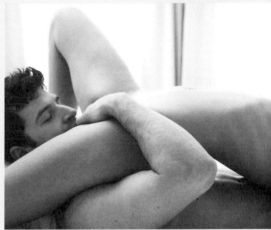

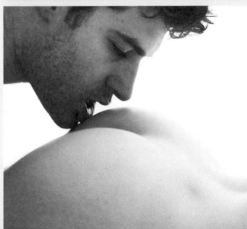

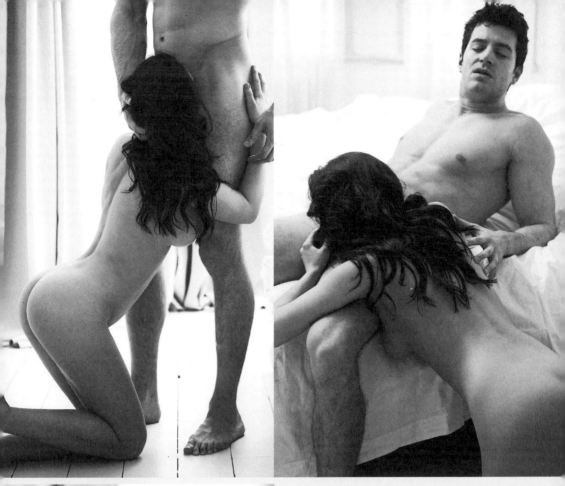

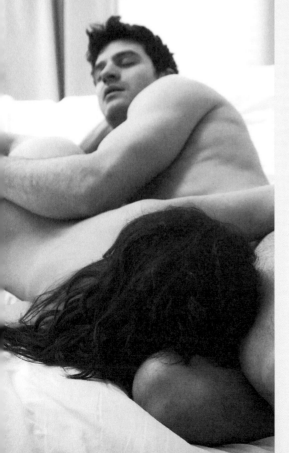

ORAL SEX FOR HIM

EXPERIMENT WITH SOME UNUSUAL ANGLES: take him in your mouth from underneath, from the side or with your head facing his feet. It will expose novel parts of his penis to the pressure of your mouth and tongue. And if your head is facing his feet, there's the added benefit that a 69 is a just a move away.

BLINDFOLD BLISS

Wearing a blindfold while you have sex can feel amazingly sensual or – depending on what you get up to – kinky. As a sex toy, it has clear advantages over the competition: unlike a vibrator, there's no chance of it running out of power. And if you don't own a blindfold, you can improvize one quickly using a silk scarf, for example. With a blindfold, you can enter the sexy world of surprise, sensuality and submission. Think of blindfolding as the extremely mild end of dominance and submission games. If you like it, you can always step things up a little (try some of the techniques in Chapter 4).

SURPRISE, SENSUALITY AND SUBMISSION

◆ Surprise: If you're wearing a blindfold, sex becomes electrifying. You only know what's happening when your lover's body is in touch with yours. As soon as your bodies break contact, you're literally in the dark about what's coming next. Will he kiss your belly, suck your toes, go down on you or something else?

◆ Sensuality: When you're deprived of sight, all your other senses become sharper. You can lose yourself in the sounds, smells, tastes and tactile sensations of sex. A friend of mine told me that her lover tastes sweeter when she kisses his body while wearing a blindfold. Enhanced sensuality applies even when you're not the one wearing a blindfold. Depriving your lover of his sight can feel liberating – you're free to look at him and marvel at his sexiness. And any inhibitions about your body vanish. You're free to help yourself.

◆ Submission: As soon as you put on a blindfold, you give up a degree of control. Your lover has the power to tease, delight or torment you as he sees fit. Yes, you can just rip off the blindfold in a second – but part of the fun of blindfolding is surrendering to your lover and being open to whatever happens. You never know – giving up control may turn out to be profoundly erotic. Alternatively, you may find it intoxicating to dominate your blindfolded partner.

BLIND WITH PASSION

The games you can play while wearing a blindfold are limited only by your imagination. Wear a blindfold and then explore your lover's body with your hands, lips and tongue. Ask him to caress you back in surprising ways, such as using a leather glove, a feather or part of his body. I like trying to work out exactly what my lover is using to touch me. When he's wearing the blindfold, deliver pleasure, then "pain". For example, kiss and lick his body, then circle his nipples with an ice cube or nibble him. Keep him guessing. Take turns to wear a blindfold during sex. I thought I'd enjoy being in charge. I was wrong – I love the freedom of surrendering. Once you start exploring, you can make all sorts of surprising discoveries about your sexual self.

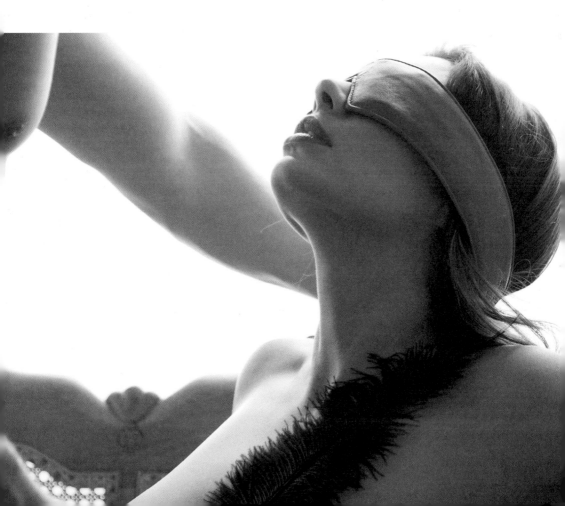

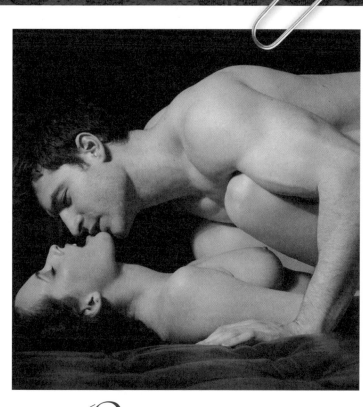

3 Orgasm

ORGASMS – YOURS AND HIS

My orgasms come in all shapes and sizes. Sometimes they're frequent; sometimes they're elusive. Sometimes they're slight and sometimes they send me flying. But the more I understand how orgasms work, the more control I seem to have over them.

SENSATIONAL SENSATIONS

It isn't absolutely necessary to orgasm every time you have sex – and sex can be a beautiful thing without climaxing. But when you're writhing with lust, an orgasm is the thing that provides that intense pleasure and that "ahhhhhh" of explosive relief.

I've discovered orgasms can come in a variety of ways: through making love or by using vibrators, hands, tongues, toes … In fact, orgasms don't even have to involve contact with the genitals. A friend of mine is lucky enough to climax through nipple stimulation alone; and some men ejaculate spontaneously when they're asleep.

Interestingly, the research I've read suggests that men and women have very similar experiences of orgasm. Back in the 1970s researchers collected students' descriptions of their orgasms. Any references to penises, vaginas and clitorises were removed, and the descriptions were then presented to a group of judges. The result? The judges couldn't tell the difference between the account of a male and a female orgasm.

For fun, ask your lover to describe his orgasms – and describe yours, too. If your descriptions are sexy enough, you may end up tearing each other's clothes off. Here's how some close friends of mine described their orgasms:

"A sudden rush – euphoria followed by deep relaxation."
"Convulsions all over my body that feel fantastic."
"An exciting build up of tension, then sudden, fast relief."
"A deep craving that I can't ignore, then deep satisfaction."
"A wave that comes and engulfs me. Time stops."

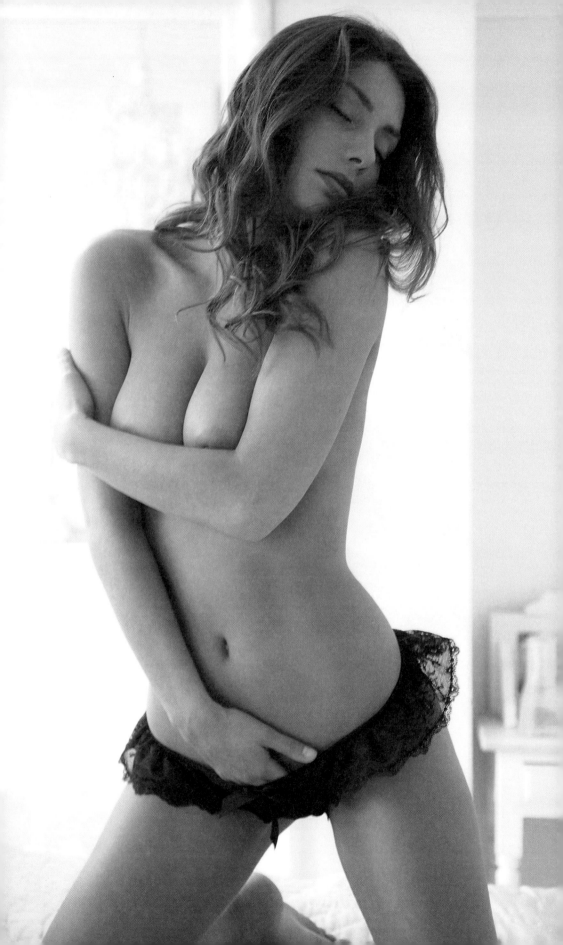

HIS ORGASM – HOW TO KNOW IT'S COMING

If you know how your lover responds sexually, you can pace yourself accordingly and slow him down if you need to (see pages 98–101). Here's what you need to know about how he climaxes:

+ Unlike women, men reach a "point of no return" – this happens a few seconds before he actually ejaculates. Once he's got to this stage, it's impossible to prevent orgasm and ejaculation (even if you withdraw all stimulation from his penis). Signs that he's reaching the point of no return are: his testicles are drawn up tightly to his body; his glans has deepened in colour; his body is tense, stiff or jerky; he's moaning uncontrollably.

+ If he's got a solid erection and droplets of pre-ejaculate on the tip of his glans, he's extremely aroused – if he's getting plenty of rhythmic stimulation on his shaft, the point of no return probably won't be far off.

+ It's possible to delay his climax, but only if you act before the point of no return. Read the delaying tactics on page 98–101.

SECRET TIP: *Ask him to go for several days without ejaculating (whether by masturbation or intercourse). His next orgasm will be much more powerful.*

YOUR ORGASM – THE BEST ROUTE

Many women have plentiful orgasms from masturbation and oral sex but find it difficult to reach orgasm during no-frills intercourse (that is, intercourse with no additional stimulation). If this applies to you, try these suggestions:

+ I wait until I'm super-excited before I have sex. Very high levels of arousal make the lower part of the vagina constrict. This creates a deliciously snug fit between me and my lover and increases my chances of having an orgasm.

+ Add frills! Depending on the sex position you're in, add

masturbation or slip a vibrating toy between your bodies (such as a pebble-shaped vibrator which makes less of a statement than a phallic one, and its curves will fit your body better).

+ Enjoy a hand-, toy- or tongue-delivered orgasm before or after sex.

+ Find out if there are any sex positions that tip you over the edge. Woman-on-top positions can help because they put you in control and you can bump and grind against his pubic bone.

+ Minimize distractions – orgasms are notoriously difficult to come by if you're preoccupied or stressed. I find it helps to get into the right headspace before I get into bed. I also try to ignore any voices in my head that say I should be trying harder, looking sexier or climaxing faster. Keep your mind busy by moaning your lover's name, gasping with pleasure or talking dirty.

SECRET TIP: *The more you hope to climax, the more elusive orgasm can become. Try reverse psychology: tell yourself you won't have an orgasm. If you don't, that's fine. If you do, it'll be relaxed and enjoyable.*

SIMULTANEOUS ORGASMS – ARE THEY WORTH IT?

Only if they happen easily! Climaxing at the same time as your lover might sound amazingly intense, but in practice it can be hard to achieve. Getting your sexual responses synchronized takes lots of communication and practice, plus it can make sex feel too goal-orientated. However, it can work well if one of you is naturally skilled at "hovering on the edge". Or, if you're lucky, your lover's orgasm may be such a turn-on that it triggers yours.

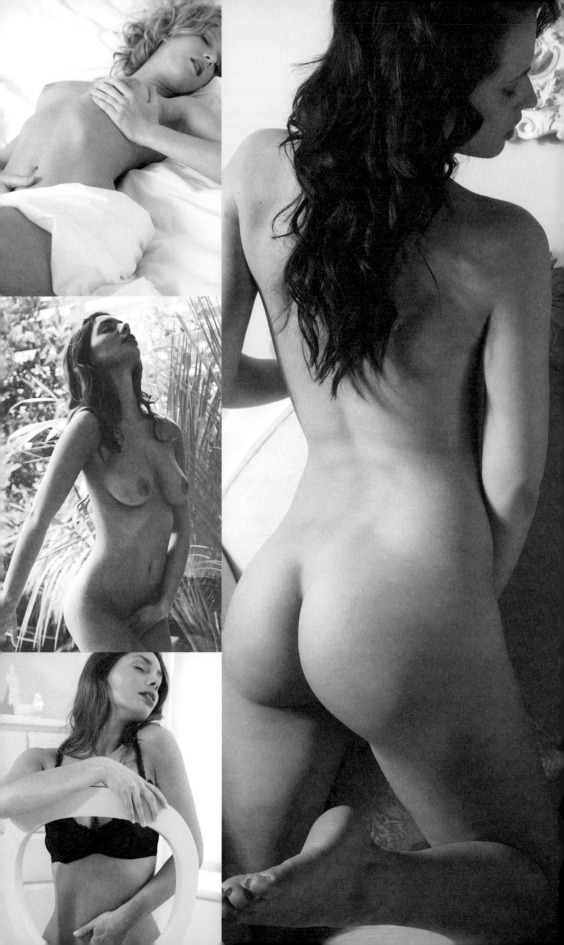

SECRETS OF ...
Masturbation

- **BREAK THE ROUTINE** Masturbate in a completely different way. Do it in an alternative position, such as standing up or sitting. Or use a new technique. Try thrusting against a pillow, rhythmically squeezing your thighs or using your "wrong" hand. I've found it's a great way to become more orgasmic in a wide variety of situations.

- **DOUBLE STIMULATION** Try massaging the clitoral head (the bud you can see) with one hand while moving your fingers or a vibrator in your vagina with the other hand. The friction will indirectly stimulate the rest of the clitoris (the invisible bit hidden inside your body), which gets stiff and erect when you're turned on.

- **TAKE A DETOUR** Turn yourself on by stroking and tweaking your inner labia before you zone in on your clitoris. These sensitive lips are often neglected, but they're rich in nerve endings.

- **DO IT MORE** Research shows masturbation increases self-esteem, sexual confidence and satisfaction levels. Women who masturbate have more orgasms with a partner. Masturbation also makes you more comfortable with your body, relieves stress and menstrual cramps, and even helps you get to sleep. What are you waiting for?

- **GO ELECTRIC** Use a vibrator. A close friend of mine who had never had an orgasm confided: "Once I found out what a vibrator orgasm was like, I learned how to get there with my hand."

- **READ ...** *Sex for One: The Joy of Self-Loving* by Betty Dodson, who's famous for her "genital show-and-tell" group masturbation sessions.

SEX ON THE EDGE

I once got my lover's attention by telling him I'd discovered a new place to have sex – somewhere that was not only super-erotic, but orgasm-friendly for both of us. Best of all, it was only a roll away from the spot where we usually made love. Once he was intrigued, I took him by the hand and led him to the bed. He looked perplexed until I positioned myself on the edge of the mattress and beckoned him over.

SPLIT-LEVEL SEX

Try these suggestions to become a convert to the joys of split-level, on-the-edge sex (experiment with sinks and counters. too):

+ You get on all fours on the edge of the bed and he enters you from a standing position. You get all the naughty thrills of the doggie position but without the hard friction on your knees. Plus, you can stimulate your clitoris while he enjoys thrusting freely from behind.
+ You stand on the floor and lean forward so your forearms are resting on the bed. He stands behind you and enters. Sex when you're both standing (or semi-standing) feels excitingly spontaneous. And you can both put your hands to creative use.
+ You lie on your back on the bed. Your bum is near the edge and your feet are flat on the floor. Then he picks up your legs and puts them wherever he wants (around his waist/a calf on each shoulder/an ankle in each hand). It's dramatic and erotic. He's sexily dominant and, if you get the height right, penetration is deep and piercing. If he needs you positioned higher, he can slide pillows under your bum.
+ He sits on the edge of the bed and you sit on his lap in a face-to-face koala hug. It feels close, intimate and sexy and you can just push him back onto the bed when you both want more freedom to move. And for an extra-special oral sex treat, get him to lie back on the bed with his bum on the edge and his feet flat on the floor. Now lavish oral attention on his penis and testicles. He can, of course, return the favour.

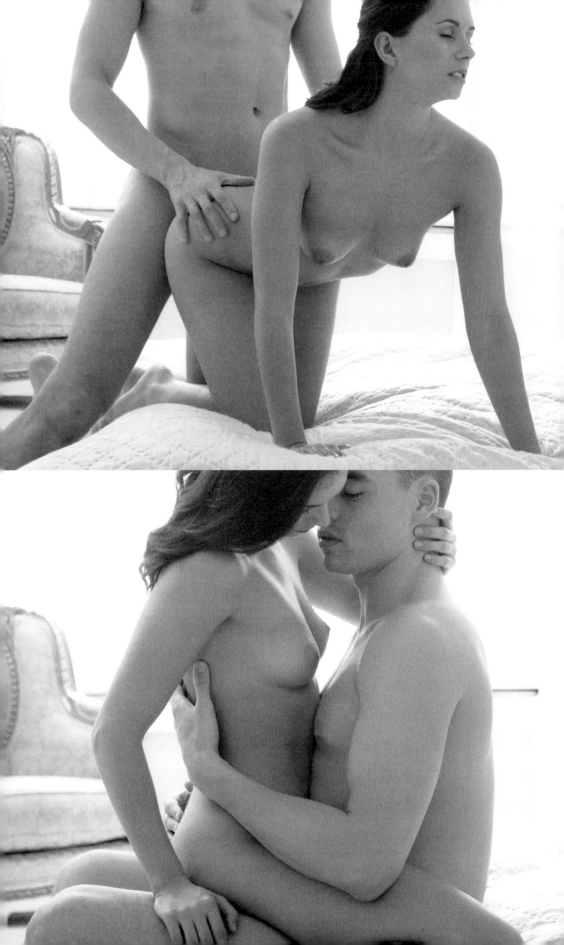

SECRET CONFESSIONS

Power games

I once asked a friend why she was so into power games with her boyfriend. She looked at me directly and said: "for the orgasms". According to her there's something about being submissive that takes arousal to new heights. And with extreme arousal comes extreme orgasm.

"I find there's something incredibly liberating about being submissive. He simply tells me what to do and I do it. Sometimes he makes his authority clear by physically restraining me. Other times, he'll threaten to spank me if I don't 'behave'. Sometimes he just uses the tone of his voice and body language. There's something thrilling about completely surrendering to someone. Being submissive makes all my normal hang-ups disappear. If he tells me to crawl across the bed on all fours, I'll happily do it. There's no thought involved – I don't think ' Should I be doing this?' I just do it. I get completely immersed in the moment and I love it.

Another great benefit of submission is that it makes me the centre of attention. People assume that if you're submissive, you're the less important partner. In fact, you're constantly in the spotlight because you're always being observed and told what to do. So being submissive makes me feel as if I'm the star of the show, but without feeling like an attention-seeking show-off. I also know that my lover is incredibly turned on by the games we play – and arousal is infectious. If I think he's getting a huge dose of pleasure, it has a knock-on effect on me. We drive each other to peaks of lust that feel addictive."

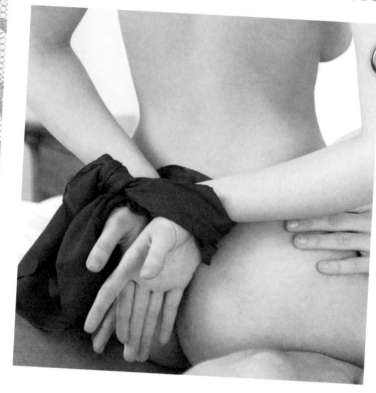

...He's in charge

WHAT'S YOUR PLEASURE?

Try this next time you have an orgasm – as you feel yourself succumbing to the ripples of pleasure, figure out exactly where they're coming from. Is the epicentre in your clitoris, the lower part of your vagina, your G-spot or higher up? Or are the sensations coming from everywhere at once?

Did you know that women can have different types of orgasm? These are clitoral orgasms, blended orgasms and uterine orgasms. Each has its own set of physical sensations, and even emotions. Once I learned about the possibilities, I had a great time experimenting to see which kinds of touch triggered which kinds of orgasm.

THE EXPLOSION – CLITORAL ORGASMS

As the name suggests, this orgasm comes from stimulating the clitoris. Most women climax this way by rubbing the clitoris with one hand (with nothing in the vagina). At the peak moment you experience intensely pleasurable feelings centred in your clitoris (I think of it as a "clitoral explosion") and the vaginal muscles contract rhythmically.

SECRET TIP: My favourite "alternative" way of having a clitoral orgasm is to direct a stream of water from the showerhead onto my clitoris as I masturbate. Wonderful!

A THRILLING COMBINATION – BLENDED ORGASMS

In my experience, blended orgasms feel less "sharp" or localized than clitoral ones, but feel more intense emotionally and take a bit longer to "come down" from. Blended orgasms happen when the clitoris and vagina, most specifically the G-spot (see page 56), are stimulated at the same time. They're sometimes called "G-spot orgasms". The few times I've had one, I've felt quite a different sensation, because both the vaginal and uterine muscles contract.

For a blended orgasm, try any of these techniques:

• Stroke your clitoris while your lover massages your G-spot by hand.

• Use a rabbit vibrator, which is designed to stimulate the clitoris and the vagina/G-spot at the same time.

• Have intercourse – the head of your lover's penis thrusts against your G-spot, while the base of his penis rubs your clitoris (or use your fingers if there's not enough penis-to-clitoris contact).

How do you know if you've had a blended orgasm? Well, you'll probably find that it feels more subtle. Read these three descriptions:

"It feels softer and slower – like my whole body is involved."

"Deep, widening and pulsating. It touches something deep in me."

"A sense of deep release that makes me feel close to my partner, but without that sudden piercing pleasure in my clitoris."

SECRET TIP: To find out if you can ejaculate, spend a long time rubbing both your clitoris and G-spot. And follow my tips on page 111.

THE BIG WHAMMY – UTERINE ORGASMS

The uterine orgasm is considered to be the most rare but most deeply satisfying orgasm. It comes about as a result of deep rapid thrusts (from a penis, hand or sex toy) that jostle the cervix high up in the vagina. During the orgasm the uterus contracts rhythmically sending deep ripples of pleasure through the whole body. A uterine orgasm is thought to be the most intensely emotional type (sometimes described as "earth-shattering"). Expect to cry, laugh or scream! And you'll probably need time to come down from the high. If you're curious about exploring uterine orgasms, you'll need to stimulate your A-spot – turn to page 56 to discover where it is and what to do with it.

SECRET TIP: Try squatting, or drawing your knees up to your chest while you lie on your back. They're not the most dignified positions but they really help your lover to discover your A-spot.

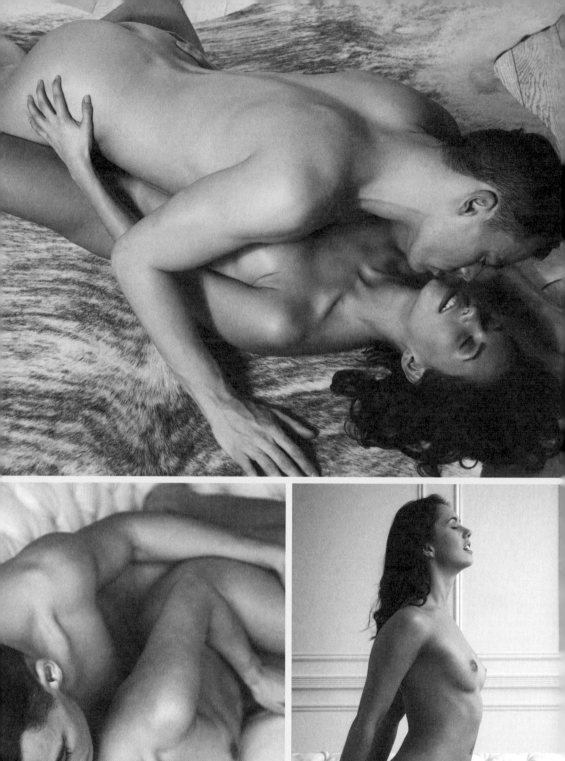
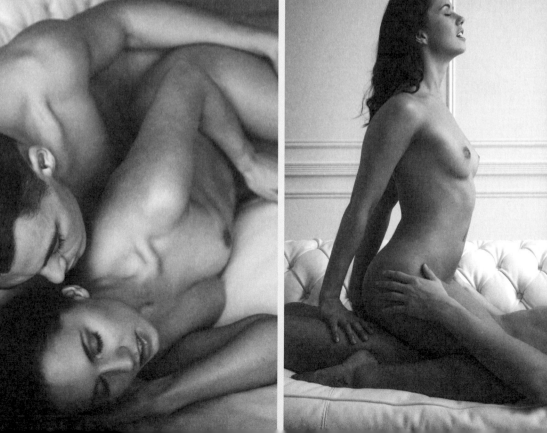

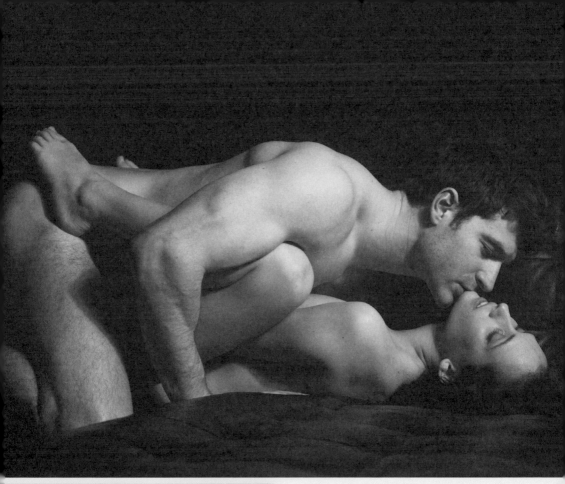

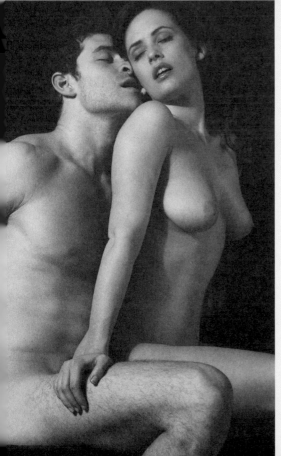

ORGASMIC SEX POSITIONS

SOME SEX POSITIONS ARE TAILOR MADE FOR ORGASM. When he's on top, pull him in tight so you get lots of orgasmic friction on your clitoris. Alternatively, pull your knees up to let him in deep (this increases the chance of a uterine orgasm; see page 91). When he lies behind you in spoons position, focus on his penis massaging your G-spot, and slip a hand between your legs. For the most orgasmic control, sit on top of him and move in the way you like best. If you find it easier to climax when you're facing away from him, simply sit on his lap in reverse.

THE SECRET GRIP

Have you ever tried lying still and making love using muscle power alone? All you need are strong pelvic floor ("PC") muscles and a willing man. In my experience, he'll be more than happy to lie back while you squeeze and pulsate him to ecstasy. And, as I've discovered, strong PC muscles bring other sexual benefits, too:

- You'll have more powerful orgasms. Orgasm is a series of muscular contractions, so, the strong muscles lead to strong contractions.
- Your vagina and G-spot will become super-sensitive. The result is more intense sensations during sex.
- You'll have a sexy new skill under your belt – one that's very useful when you want to have extremely discreet sex (see page 136).

SECRET TIP: *Get him to flex his PC muscles during sex too. If you both do it at the same time, it feels incredibly erotic.*

TEST YOUR MUSCLE POWER

First, you need to know what and where your PC muscles are, and how strong or weak they are. Some quick anatomy: "PC" stands for "pubococcygeal", and PC muscles run from your pubic bone to your tailbone, supporting all the bits in between, such as your clitoris, urethra, vagina, perineum and anus. Imagine you want to stop yourself from peeing – tense those muscles. You should be able to find them instantly (your lover can find his in this way, too).

To test your muscle tone, insert a finger into your vagina and contract your PC muscles. How strongly squeezed is your finger? A vice-like grip is a sign of super-strong PC muscles; and a medium-to-firm squeeze suggests your PC muscles are in good shape. If you can't feel anything, or only a mild squeeze, you'll gain a lot of benefits from the PC workout, opposite.

SECRET TIP: *I love this fun way of testing your PC muscles: peel a banana and slide it into your vagina (use lube). If you can "chop" it in half with your muscles, you're definitely pretty strong down there!*

MY PERSONAL PC WORKOUT

When you're new to PC muscle exercises (also known as Kegel exercises after the doctor who invented them), you might find it easier or more comfortable to do them lying down. Follow these steps:

+ Lie on your back on the bed/floor with your knees bent. Imagine that your lover is inside you and you're trying to grip his penis hard. Squeeze your vaginal muscles tight (but keep your abdominal muscles and the rest of your body relaxed). Hold the squeeze for at least four seconds, then relax completely. Repeat this five times in a row and try to do it three times a day.
+ When you're used to the exercises, do them standing up and sitting down – in fact in any place or at any time that you think of them. Work up to a series of 10 contractions, three times every day.

A SEX WORKOUT

It can take a while to build up strong PC muscles – weeks rather than days – but don't let that stop you experimenting with muscle techniques straight away during sex. In fact, treat sex as another opportunity to do your workout. Try any of these moves on his shaft:

+ Repeated fast or slow squeezes.
+ Gripping him for as long as you can, then slowly relaxing.
+ Gentle pulsing, fluttering or rippling.
+ A hard, tight squeeze just before he climaxes.

Another technique you can try is the "secret language", pioneered by teachers of Tantric sex. You give him a slow squeeze and he flexes his penis slowly in response. Then you give him three fast squeezes and he gives you three fast flexes. Think of it as a "conversation" between your genitals.

SECRET TIP: *I find muscle squeezes most titillating in sex positions where I'm on top but don't have much freedom to move. For example, when he sits on the floor and I sit facing him on his lap.*

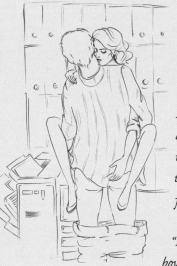

SECRET CONFESSIONS

Sex at work

I've had sex in some unusual places, but never at work. I've always been curious to find out what the appeal of this particular venue is. Is it just the thrill of being caught? These are some of my favourite explanations:

"I'm the keyholder to my office and sometimes my boyfriend comes to meet me at work when everyone else has gone home. We've often had standing-up sex with me leaning over the edge of my desk. I like it because it feels so wrong! I've spent all day being good, polite and professional, and sex in the office is a reversal of all that. It's a bit like the moment when the prim secretary takes off her glasses, lets her hair down and shows everyone what she's really like!"

"High-tech office chairs are great for sex – the ones where you can adjust the height and tilt really far back."

"I met my boyfriend at work and we had to keep our relationship a secret in case it was frowned upon. But we took every opportunity to be naughty when we were out of sight – I gave him blowjobs in the stationery cupboard and we had sex in the toilet and even on the fire escape. I'm sure other people do the same – offices are melting pots of sexual tension."

"I once seduced my boyfriend after work and we had sex on my boss's desk. The sex was amazing, and it felt particularly naughty because I had a bit of a crush on my boss at the time."

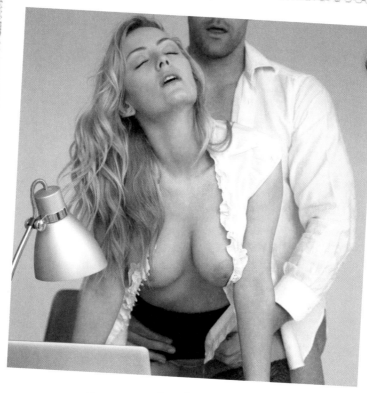

... A good day at the office

SLOWING HIM DOWN

To keep sex unpredictable, I like to vary its length: sometimes a thrilling quickie; sometimes an average-sized romp; and sometimes an evening of slow-burning passion. If your lover excels at the quickies but not the slow-burners, you'll be pleased to know there are some sexy and effective secrets for delaying his orgasm.

HOW NOT TO DELAY ORGASM

The desire to delay orgasm is so common that a multi-million pound business has built up around it. There are creams, lotions and pills that promise to help men to last longer. The problem is that they usually numb sensation. So, although your lover may successfully delay his orgasm, sex becomes less pleasurable, sensual and fun. The same problem applies to other methods of desensitizing the penis, such as wearing an extra-thick condom or two condoms at once. And if your lover tries to lower his arousal levels by thinking about something unsexy, such as work deadlines, it may well have an effect, but with the danger that he'll lose interest completely.

Some men rely on alcohol to last longer. Alcohol slows down all bodily reflexes including ejaculation, but with the following drawbacks: he won't be as fully present or focused during sex; he may need to drink more over time to get the same effect; dependency on alcohol can be hard to break; and if he drinks too much, it can be difficult for him to get an erection or to ejaculate at all.

SECRET TIP: *Never complain that he's too quick – criticism may destroy his confidence. Be positive. I once said to a boyfriend, "I love feeling you inside me – I want to keep you there longer."*

THE QUICK-FIX SOLUTION

On the opposite page, I describe a tried-and-trusted method of delaying orgasm that works permanently – but it takes practice. If you want a quick-fix, try the squeeze technique. It won't turn your lover into a long-distance runner but it can help in highly charged situations. The squeeze technique was developed by sex researchers Masters and Johnson. When your lover is close to coming (see page 82), place your thumb on his frenulum and your index and middle finger on the other side of his penis (just underneath the ridge). Now squeeze firmly for three to four seconds. His erection will wilt slightly and he'll feel less close to climaxing. If you're having sex and he doesn't want to pull out, try this handy variation – your lover simply reaches down and gives his shaft a firm squeeze at the base.

SECRET TIP: *Gently tugging his testicles downward can also help him to last longer (they contract and pull in tight to his body when he's close to coming). This won't hurt him, but it's worth warning him you're going to do it!*

TAKING CONTROL

The true secret of delaying climax is for him to learn ejaculatory control. Like riding a bike, ejaculatory control is a skill he'll have for life. The first thing he'll need to know – and you can help him – is exactly how aroused he is at any one moment, not just roughly, but exactly: using a scale of one to ten, with one being "not turned on at all" and ten being "ejaculation and orgasm".

Most importantly, he needs to learn when he's reaching level eight or nine, which is the point of ejaculatory inevitability (this is the stage where he's about to lose control – even if all stimulation stops, he'll come anyway – see page 82). To try the following exercise, you'll both need to feel fairly relaxed talking about sex. And, in the nicest possible way, you'll need to broach the subject of slowing him down. Start by telling him you've got a suggestion that would make your sex life even better. One that would maximize your pleasure and be great for him too ... Try to make your tone light-hearted, playful and suggestive rather than serious and earnest.

Once you've got your lover on board, explain mischievously that you'll need to give him lots of oral sex and hand caresses (a great incentive for most men). Then settle down to an evening of playing around and experimenting – stroke his penis with your hands, pump it, lick the shaft and glans with your tongue, enclose him in your mouth and tickle his testicles with your fingertips. As you do this, ask him to give you a running commentary of how aroused he is from one to ten. When he reaches the higher end of the scale, stop stimulating him. Don't start again until he's used one or more of the techniques below to get back in control.

SLOWING DOWN TECHNIQUES

+ The PC squeeze (see pages 94–5) – like women, men have PC muscles. You can help him to locate his by placing two fingers just behind his testicles and asking him to squeeze (as if he were trying to stop the flow of pee). When he reaches an eight in the arousal scale (see above), tell him to squeeze his PC muscles hard for several seconds. Some men prefer to do two or three medium squeezes or several quick, light ones – whatever does the job is fine. Think of PC muscle squeezes as the brakes on a car. They do a great job of slowing him down and they work quickly too.

+ Full-body relaxation – as your partner ascends the arousal scale, you'll probably notice his breathing gets shallower and his body gets more tense and rigid. When he tells you he's getting as high as a seven or an eight, ask him to relax his body. Encourage him by stroking his belly, chest or shoulders and taking several deep, calm breaths in time with him. This should stop his arousal zooming up to a nine or a ten.

+ Switching focus – this is a mental trick that your partner can do when he hits the high scores. It's simple: instead of thinking about the sensations in his penis, he switches his focus to another part of his body. The best places to pick are those where the sensations feel good, but not orgasmic; for example, his inner thighs, his belly, his testicles or his perineum. Sometimes it may simply be enough to switch his focus from the head of the penis to the base.

When he's super-skilled at pinpointing the high points of his arousal and getting himself back down to, say, a five, a six or a seven, he won't even need you to stop stimulating him. Then he can start applying his skills to sex.

SECRET TIP: *Even if he's a master of ejaculation, he can still use the one to ten rating for fun. It's funny and sexy when my lover shouts "Oh god, that's a ten!" And when he's doing something fantastic to me, I rate him, too.*

SPEEDING HIM UP

Sometimes men have the opposite problem – they're very slow to come or they can't come at all. If this affects your lover, it's worth him getting a medical checkup, because there are some health problems that delay or prevent ejaculation. If there's no underlying problem, the chances are that he's got something on his mind – perhaps he's sexually self-conscious, fearful of losing control or worried about getting you pregnant. Perhaps it's got nothing to do with sex – maybe he's distracted by work problems or he's feeling depressed or anxious. Apart from encouraging him to talk about his feelings, make sure that he's fully relaxed before you make love. Try the massage on pages 44–7. It's also a good idea to get him as aroused as possible before sex – try some of the techniques over the page.

FAST-TRACK ORGASM

Although long, lingering sex sessions are fantastic, I don't always have time for them. That's why it's good to know some quick routes to orgasm. I've noticed that fast, intense orgasms (mine and his) are often triggered by a sudden and unexpected thrill. The trick is do something genuinely surprising – and something extremely sexy.

A FEAST FOR HIS EYES

Men love visual surprises because their arousal levels are closely linked to what they see. All of the following may be titillating for you, too:

+ Swallow your inhibitions and masturbate in front of him. Lie back and show him exactly how you turn yourself on. Close your eyes, arch your back and lick your lips as you start to lose control.
+ Do an erotic dance around a chair. I've found a chair enables me to do all sorts of naughty moves, from straddling it with my legs open to bending over to expose my bum. Read the steps on page 30–31.
+ This is another favourite technique of mine – slip into a tight white T-shirt and panties and surprise him by joining him in the shower – get wet while you're kissing him. He'll love your impulsiveness, *and* he'll love the way your wet T-shirt and panties cling to your body.
+ Men like genital close ups – he'll love it if you greet him in bed with your legs apart. Or adopt a sex position you want to try – before he enters the bedroom.

PERSONALITY CHANGE

Get a rush by doing the opposite of what you usually do. If you tend to initiate sex, withdraw completely. When he tries to embrace you, say "no way" with a wicked glint in your eye. Or, if you're usually "too tired", drag him to bed and ravish him like a sex kitten.

If you normally dedicate yourself to his pleasure in bed, become selfish – demand his tongue, lips and hands on your hotspots. Or if you're usually the one to call the shots, turn into his sex slave.

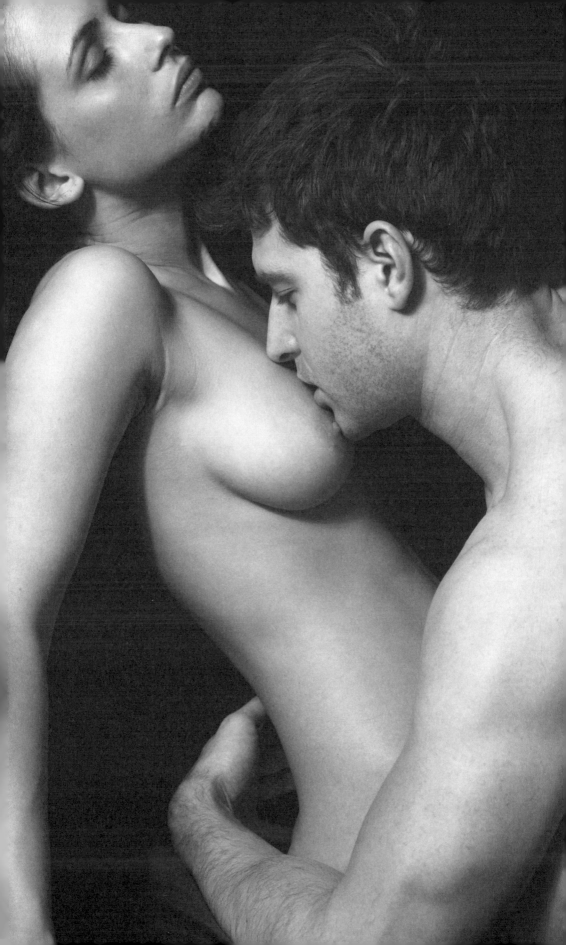

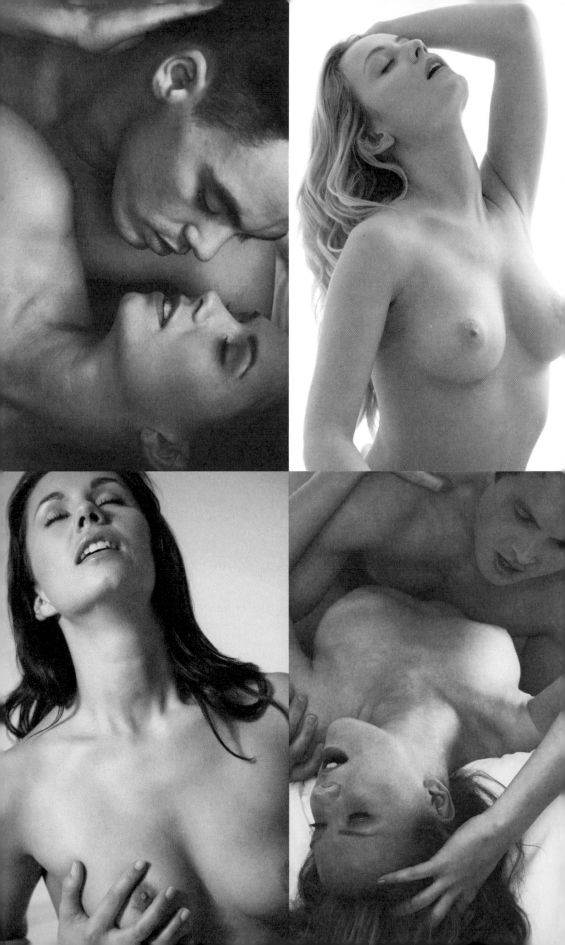

SECRETS OF ...

Enhancing orgasm

◆ **USE THE STOP-START TECHNIQUE** Each time you feel yourself getting close to orgasm, stop all stimulation, and take some long, deep, belly breaths. This will take you back to a plateau of arousal – now work your way back up to a state of high excitement. Repeat this stop–start process until you can't bear it any longer – then surrender to an intense orgasm.

◆ **BE SELFISH (OR SELFLESS)** Sometimes I like dedicating an entire sex session to my orgasm or to his orgasm, but not to both. This way we each get all the attention and focus we need.

◆ **TARGET THE HOTSPOTS** Single out his P-spot and F-spot (see page 59) as he builds up to orgasm. Ask him to concentrate on your G-spot and A-spot, too (see page 56).

◆ **RELAX, RELAX, RELAX** Consciously relax your PC muscles (see pages 94–5) so you're not holding even the tiniest bit of tension in your genitals (think of the level of relaxation you need to pee). I've found that having sex in this profound state of relaxation always gives me incredible orgasms.

◆ **GIVE HIM THE LOOK OF LOVE** To achieve the maximum in soul-baring intensity, try to hold your lover's gaze for the duration of your (and his) orgasm.

◆ **FOCUS ON THE DETAILS ...** The tingling in your thighs and genitals, and the melting sensation in your belly. When I do this, the small sensations come together in a big, glorious crescendo.

THE ART OF THE QUICKIE

Whenever I want to feel desirable, wicked and wanton, I suggest a quickie to my lover. It's a great way of reviving the heady, lust-driven early days of our relationship. And although it may not be the most intimate sex we ever have, the pay-off is the naughty glow that lingers for hours afterwards.

THREE QUICKIE SECRETS

Here are three facts that might challenge what you think about quickies:

+ One: you don't have to be in a red-hot relationship to have a quickie. In fact, you can even use quickies as a form of sex therapy if your lovemaking has taken a nosedive. People tend to think if sex has slipped down their list of priorities, they should coax it back up with long sessions and soul-merging romance. Sometimes the opposite is true – fast and furious sex gets you back in the running without putting you under too much pressure. I've found if I haven't had sex for a while, a quickie session is a great way to kick start my sex life again.

+ Two: quickies can be romantic. Especially if you gaze into each other's eyes all the way through. And especially if you call each other later on to say: "I love you – that was fantastic."

+ Three: you don't have to be turned on before you embark on a quickie. It often works to throw yourself into the action and trust your body to respond. The passionate urgency of quickies may be enough to arouse you.

SECRET TIP: *Give him super-fast fellatio of no more than 10–15 strokes. It'll not only get him hot, it'll make him wet enough to ensure a smooth entry.*

WORK TO A DEADLINE

The best quickies are when you've got only a tiny window of opportunity. Try this: initiate sex when you've got a set-in-stone deadline. For example: a train you have to catch; the arrival of his parents for dinner; the school run; or a meeting to attend. As well as focusing your body and mind on the task, a deadline makes you more excited than usual. Part of the reason is anxiety: your fight or flight response gets switched on, resulting in an adrenaline high. Your heart starts pounding, you breathe faster, your cheeks get flushed and everything feels more intense than usual. One of my most thrilling quickies was in a train compartment. We could hear the ticket collector coming toward us shouting "tickets please".

SECRET TIP: *Try this five-minute sex schedule: one minute on kissing and foreplay; three minutes on sex; and one minute on making yourself presentable again.*

QUICK STARTS

Men love being propositioned – a request for quickie sex will almost always put a smile on his face. Even the way you initiate a quickie is likely to be a huge turn-on. Try any of these:

+ Whisper a filthy proposition in his ear.
+ Push him against a wall and kiss him hard.
+ As he bends to kiss you goodbye (when you're lying in bed), pull him on top.
+ Guide his hand under your dress/skirt so he can discover you're not wearing any panties.
+ Go up to him at a party, fix him with a wicked look then drag him to the bathroom.
+ Catch him at the front door. Say you won't let him past until you've had your way with him.
+ Keep it simple. Say: "I want you … *now.*"

- Text him an instruction to meet you in the bedroom/boardroom/ stairwell/stationery cupboard/lift in 60 seconds.
- Join him for his morning shower and start groping him.
- Meet his gaze, then kiss him while undoing his belt.

SECRET TIP: *Men's testosterone levels are highest in the morning – so pounce on him first thing.*

SEXY MIDDLES

There's no time for niceties in quickie sex. If you're going to go down on him – or him on you – pull his penis out of his trousers and go for it. And as soon as he's hard and you're wet, take the minimum of clothes off (ideally, just your panties) and slip him inside you.

Choose the position that allows you both to reach a fast climax. He'll need to thrust freely and you may need hand-room to stimulate your clitoris. Standing rear-entry positions are good – just find a nearby desk, table or other surface to lean on. Alternatively, sit on a counter, table or car bonnet and pull him between your legs.

I tend to throw in more kinkiness than I usually would. It adds to the sense of wildness and can get you to the peak quicker. Talk dirty to speed things up.

HAPPY ENDINGS

If you reach a climactic ending, you'll probably have a couple of minutes to stare cross-eyed at each other before you compose yourselves. However, if you don't reach the finishing line, you can follow up with some lightning handwork (from you or him); agree to continue later; or get dressed, straighten your hair and let the sexual charge fuel you though the day.

Don't speak after quickie sex – just communicate with eye contact and naughty grins. If one of you has to leave, say goodbye with a passionate kiss and no words.

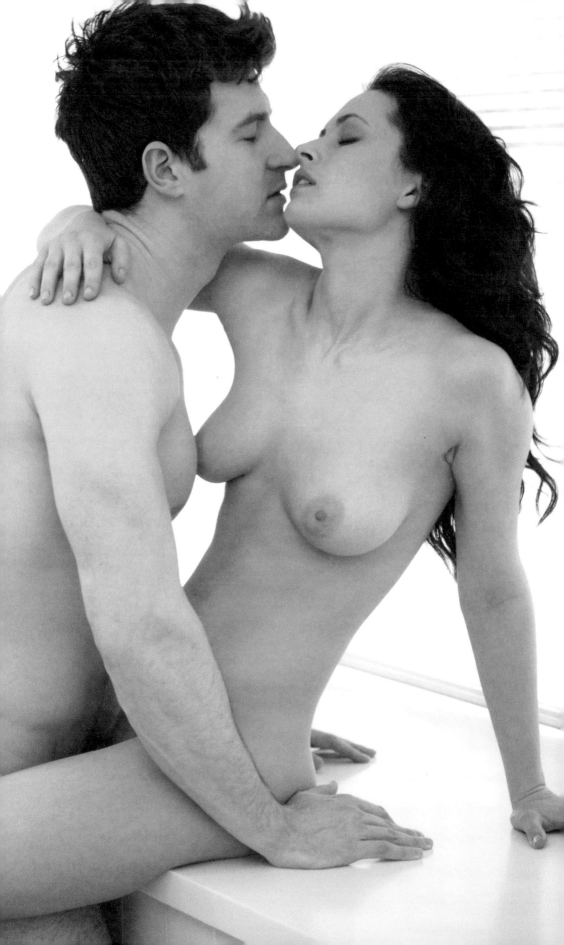

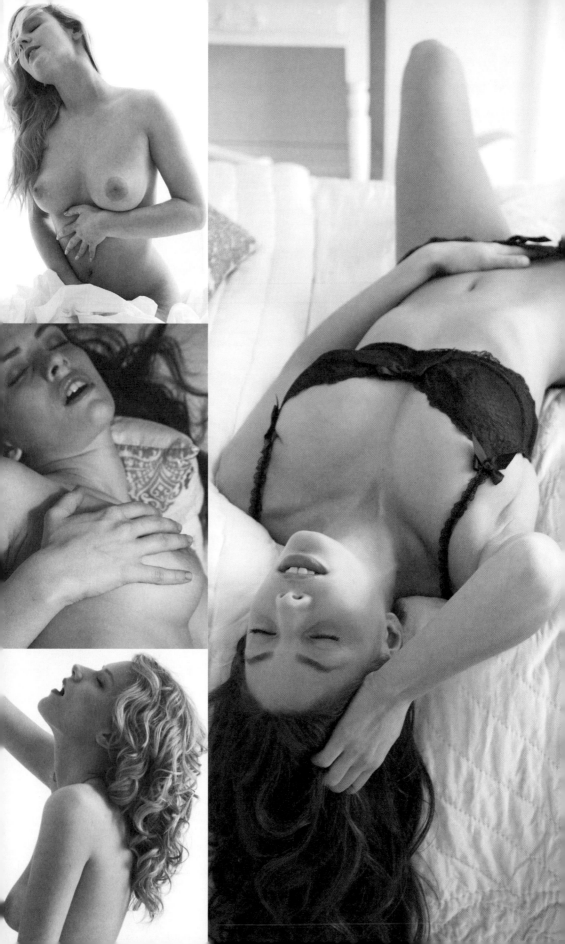

SECRETS OF ...

Female ejaculation

♦ **BELIEVE IT'S POSSIBLE** Explore your body with an "anything-could-happen" mindset.

♦ **LIE BACK AND RELAX** Aim for really deep relaxation that allows you to shed your inhibitions and abandon yourself to pure eroticism. The biggest block to ejaculating is fear of letting go. It's advisable to empty your bladder completely as this helps you to relax, and if you do ejaculate, you can be sure it's not urine.

♦ **GO G-SPOTTING** Ejaculation happens during G-spot stimulation so you'll need a very hands-on relationship with yours. If you can't find your G-spot (see page 56) with your fingers, invest in a G-spotter (a dildo or vibrator with a curved or bulbous end). If you can find your G-spot with your fingers, rub it firmly in small circular movements. Keep going even if it feels weird. Soon your G-spot will get larger and change in texture. Now just keep going ...

♦ **DOUBLE THE PLEASURE** Use your index finger to gently stroke or tickle your clitoris while your other hand massages your G-spot. If this sounds like too much multi-tasking, ask your lover to help.

♦ **PUSH!** When you're close to coming, remove your fingers and push down/let go as if you're trying to pee. This will make you ejaculate if you're going to. If it doesn't work the first time, keep alternating G-spot stimulation with pushing down.

♦ **BE STRONG** If you've got strong pelvic floor muscles, you're more likely to ejaculate. Do the PC workout on page 95, starting now.

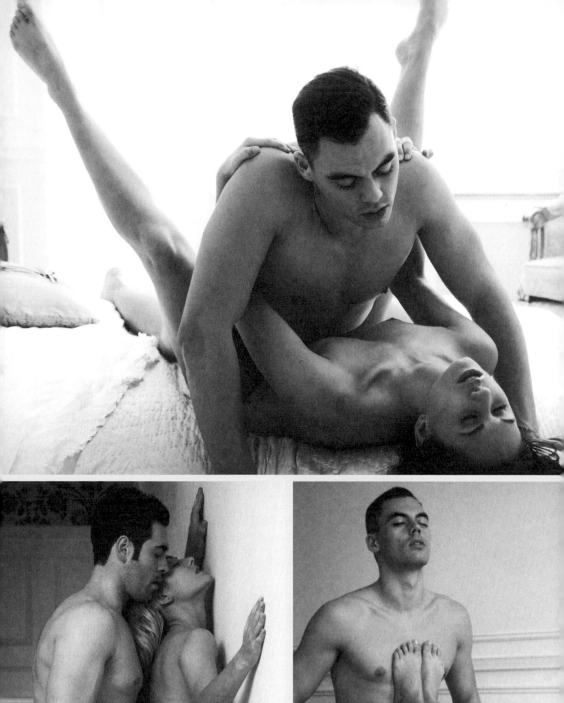
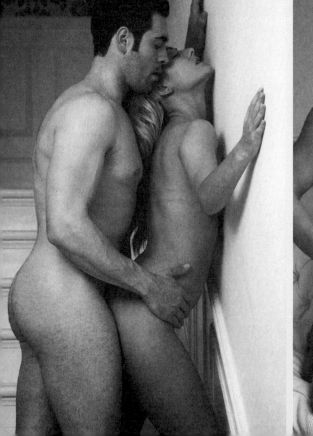
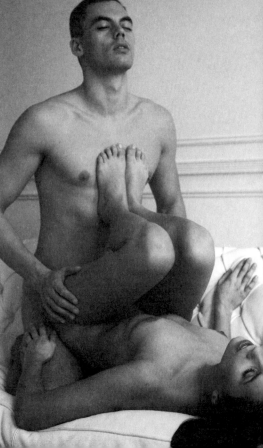

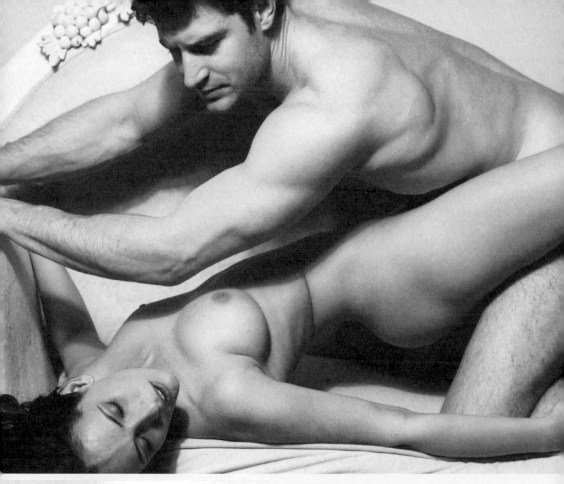

ORGASMIC X-RATED SEX POSITIONS

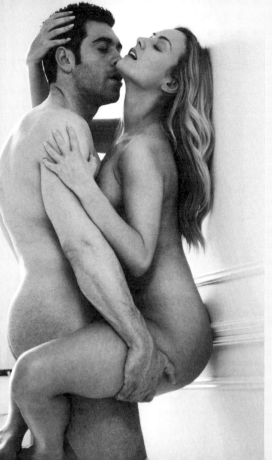

SOMETIMES SEX IN A NAUGHTY POSITION is just what you need to take you over the edge. Sex while standing up always feels thrilling, but you can make it even more X-rated by doing it pressed up against a wall (especially if he picks you up). You can make man-on-top positions extra erotic by opening your legs in a wide "V", by pushing your hips in the air or by pulling your knees to your breasts.

THE ORGASM DIET

It's surprising but true: one of the best ways of improving orgasms for both you and your lover is to stop having them. I think of it as an orgasm diet. You don't have to give up sexual intimacy – the opposite, in fact. The whole idea of the orgasm diet is that you go back to the basics of intimacy and rediscover each other. Imagine being able to turn the clock back to when you were both inexperienced teenagers with a burning desire to explore …

Whenever I've gone on an orgasm diet, it's had a miraculous effect on my sex life, making it more erotic, passionate and sensual. The orgasm diet is a series of four sensual sessions in which you start with touch and then build up to sex. You can space the four sessions over four nights, over a week, a fortnight or longer. If you and your lover enjoy one of the sessions in particular, you can repeat it as many times as you like.

SECRET TIP: Make a box of erotic toys (see page 128) to keep near your bed. My favourite is a peacock feather – it's sexy and decadent and I love lying on my front while my lover strokes my back with it.

BEFORE YOU START

Make the following pact with your lover before you begin. Agree to:

+ Wait until your fourth session before you have an orgasm together.
+ Only do things that feel pleasurable/fun/sensual. Stop if anything feels like hard work.
+ Take away any performance pressure – there's no obligation for either of you to do anything. You don't have to get aroused, and your lover doesn't have to get (or keep) an erection. You don't have to impress or please each other.
+ Relax during each session so that you're fully "present". Give yourself up to all the sensations. If your mind wanders, bring it back to what you're feeling in your body.

SESSION ONE

Start by canoodling. Pretend that you're learning to touch each other for the first time, with one important rule: you mustn't touch each other's genitals and nipples. If it helps, imagine you're a couple of virginal teenagers.

Experiment with different types of touch: nibble each other's earlobes; have a steamy kissing session; snuggle up against each other; kiss each other's toes; run your hands over each other's bum; lick a patch of skin and blow on it; caress each other with a silk scarf. Use your toes, fingers, hair, legs, lips and tongue as stroking tools. Talk to each other – say what feels good, or just go "mmmmm…"

SECRET TIP: Discover the sexiness of making out with your underwear on. Tease him by slipping your fingers under the waistband of his boxers. Let your hand linger for a few moments, then pull back.

SESSION TWO

In this session, get a bit more daring – carry on exploring like you did last time, but include genitals and nipples. Let yourselves get turned on, but don't climax. Let arousal come and go – if he gets an erection, just include it in your explorations. If you want to give him oral sex, make it relaxed and pleasurable – for example, keep your mouth and tongue soft and find a comfortable position where he can stroke you at the same time. And get him to touch you in new ways, for example, his flat palm pressed against your vulva or a slow line traced from your clitoris to your vagina. If you want something in particular, ask.

SECRET TIP: Men often don't admit they love their nipples being played with. Try licking the tip of your finger and drawing slow circles around each of his nipples. Ask him how it feels.

SESSION THREE

Do the same as you've done in the previous two sessions, but with one major difference: when you're both aroused climb on top of him and slide his penis inside you. Rather than doing the usual in-out, grinding and rubbing movements of intercourse, just stay still or move very gently together. Savour the sensations, but don't let them build up to a peak. Experiment with the secret grip (see pages 94–5) and stroke each other's face, chest or belly to keep the focus on sensuality. If his erection disappears, it's fine because climax isn't your aim. Keep telling each other what feels good.

SECRET TIP: *When you're sitting astride him, take his hands and pull him up into a sitting position. Wrap your arms around his body and treat him to a deeply passionate kiss.*

SESSION FOUR

This time you can both go as far as having an orgasm. Condense all the three previous steps into a single experience, building up gradually so that your route to climax is slow, sensual and meandering. Let orgasm happen by any method: his fingers caressing your G-spot; your mouth caressing his penis; oral sex in the 69 position; or the rhythmic rocking of intercourse. And if orgasm doesn't come naturally, don't make it into a goal – just let it happen (or not). Remember that your only aim is pleasure.

Rather than going back to "normal" sex after the orgasm diet, remember the sensual lessons you've learned and keep applying them. And repeat the orgasm diet whenever you feel like it, but particularly when you want to rediscover each other sexually.

SECRET TIP: *You may find you're so orgasm-hungry at the end of your diet, you'll be able to come in a completely different way from usual. Try experimenting. My lover managed to give me an orgasm using just his toe!*

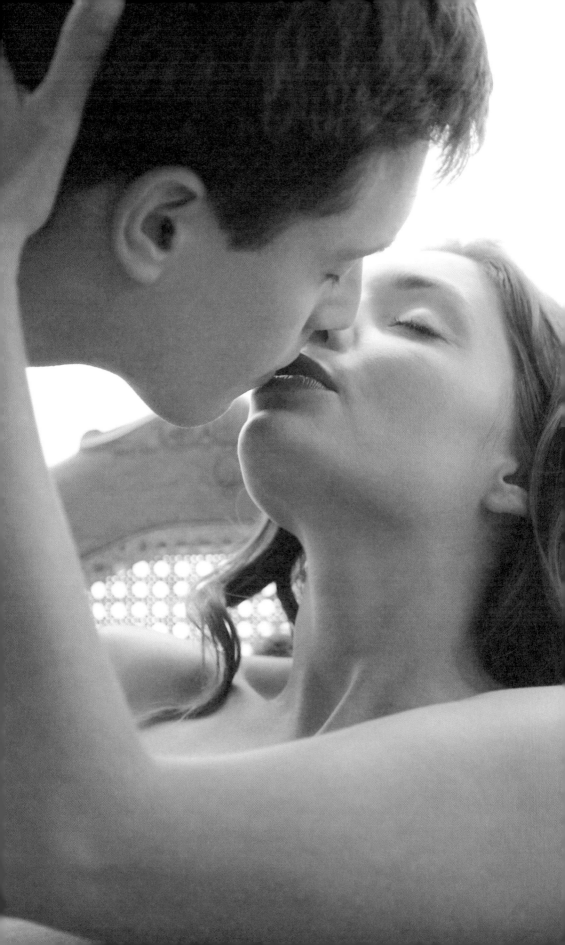

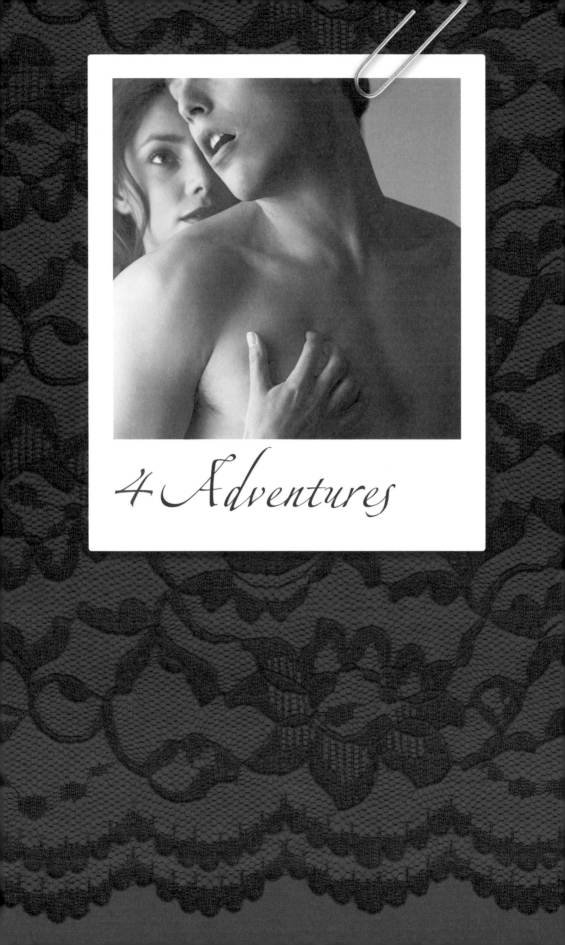

4 Adventures

SEX DARES

If you haven't left your sexual comfort zone recently, I recommend playing sex dares. I've always found it a great way to shake up my sex life, and I love thinking up naughty things I can do with my lover. Once you start playing it, you'll find it addictive. And your lover will enjoy the buzz of trying new things in bed.

PLAYING THE GAME

The preparation is all part of the fun – especially if you've never sat down with your lover and openly discussed your fantasies. Get two blank pieces of paper. You're each going to write down a list of sex dares or "sexcapades" in the following three categories: "Easy", "Full-on" and "I couldn't possibly do that ... or could I?"

Be creative – think about things you've always wanted to try, things you've read about or past erotic acts. Think of sex as part of your life where you can let your hair down and be playful – don't be embarrassed to suggest something. Your list might start like this:

• Easy: have a Brazilian wax; let him give me oral sex outdoors; do a dirty dancing routine for him; act out a scene from an erotic movie.
• Full-on: have webcam sex; have sex on a swing; describe in blow-by-blow detail how I like to pleasure myself – then demonstrate; try a standing-up 69; play kinky doctor and nurse ...
• I couldn't possibly do that ... or could I? Reveal a really kinky fantasy; make a sex film; have anal sex; be a dominatrix.

When you've exhausted your erotic imagination, swap lists and have fun reading each other's suggestions. Cut up your dares and allocate them to three piles according to their easiness level (if you disagree about which category a dare should go in, put it in the harder category).

Next, nominate a night of the week as "dare night" – and stick to it each week. On the dare night randomly pluck a slip of paper from the easy pile. You can work up to the "I couldn't possiblys" in the coming weeks – you'll be an experienced dare devil by then.

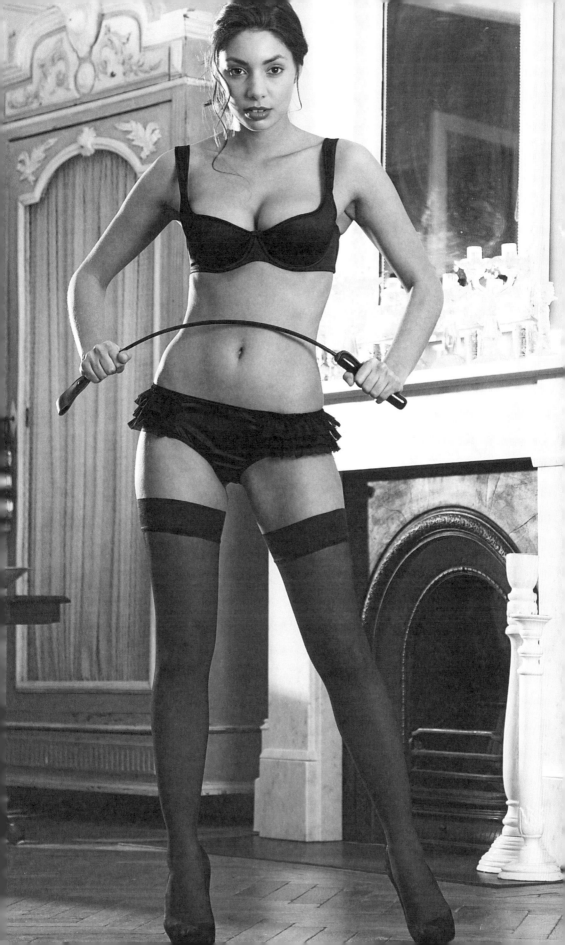

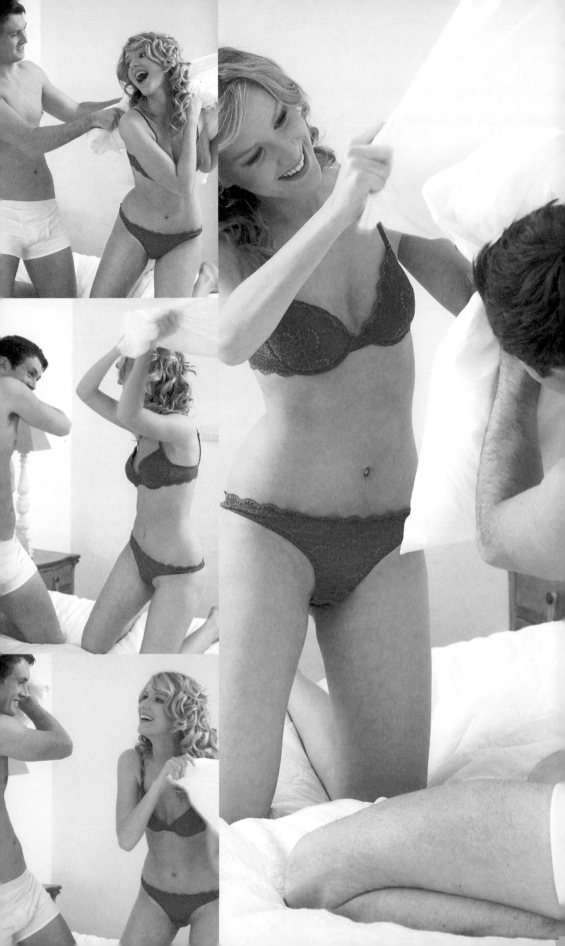

SECRETS OF ...
Adult playtime

+ **INVENT A NEW SEX POSITION** ... and give it an unlikely name. Then discuss it with your lover innocently in front of friends: "Hey, do you fancy a chai latte when we get home?"

+ **GET INTO A FIGHT** I love pillow fights that turn sexy. When you've beaten him into submission, pin his arms behind his head and climb victoriously on top.

+ **HAVE ANIMAL SEX** He's a lion, you're a kitten, or vice versa.

+ **TRY NAKED YOGA** Do a shoulderstand and ask him to give you oral sex. Prepare for a head rush.

+ **69 WITH A TWIST** Get into a side-by-side 69 position. Now instead of licking each other's genitals, suck each other's toes.

+ **HAVE FOOD SEX** Smother each other in anything sticky, runny, creamy ... When you can't get any messier, press your bodies together.

+ **MAKE UP A SEX RULE** And he has to obey it for the night. For example, no hands, only tongues; or standing sex only.

+ **WOW HIM WITH A NEW HAIRSTYLE** Buy a pubic hair stencil and wax your pubes into a heart or diamond shape. Or make your bare skin look gorgeous with stick-on crystals designed for this area.

+ **PLAY SEXY HIDE AND SEEK** Each hiding place becomes the venue for a naughty foreplay act.

BEYOND THE BEDROOM

Want to know a secret that will instantly transform your sex life? Give up having sex in bed. For me, moving sex out of the bedroom has always added a frisson of naughtiness – and, often, a thrilling challenge. It makes for great sex in other ways too:

+ It forces me and my lover into some sexy teamwork.
+ It makes me discover the raunchy joys of sex positions that just don't work on a mattress – standing doggy, for example.
+ It gives me some unforgettable sexy memories.

IS THIS SEAT TAKEN?

Chair sex is one of the first joys you'll discover when you get frisky away from the bed. It feels wickedly impromptu, and it means you can assume delicious erotic control by straddling him and bouncing up and down. And he gets passionately pumped as he sits back and admires the view.

SECRET TIP: If you want to try something kinky with your lover, get him to sit on a dining room chair, then tie his wrists and ankles to the chair legs. Now you're free to give him a blowjob or sit on his lap, whatever takes your fancy.

IN THE DRIVING SEAT

Having sex in a car is an exciting homage to adolescent lust. Play romantic or raunchy music – anything that matches your mood. And always park somewhere completely legal, with no one around for miles.

SECRET TIP: Have sex on the car instead of in it. Use the car bonnet in the same way you'd use a kitchen counter (read on!). For extra naughtiness, lie back on the bonnet and ask him to give you oral first.

GOING WILD IN THE GARDEN

Slipping outside for an erotic tryst in the garden can make sex feel both risqué and romantic. If your garden is heavily overlooked, wait until it's completely dark, take cover in a pop-up tent or follow the "invisibility" tips on page 136.
SECRET TIP: *Have sex on a tree – look for low boughs you can sit on, sturdy trunks to lean on; or branches to hang off.*

IF YOU CAN'T STAND THE HEAT …

Sex in the kitchen offers the fantastic benefit of wicked and wanton counter sex. I love the drama of knocking the dishes aside in urgent lust, then brazenly jumping onto the counter, leaning back and pulling him in deep. Men love this position because it gives them the ability to thrust freely while standing with no weight to support.
SECRET TIP: *Try this for achingly deep and sensual penetration: instead of letting your legs hang off the counter, put your heels on the edge and pull your knees into your chest. Now guide him into you.*

HOT 'N' WET

Getting jiggy in the shower is sensual bliss – picture jets of water bouncing off you, steam caressing your bodies, fingers gliding over wet curves. My favourite position for shower sex is standing doggy – you lean forward and press your hands against the wall; he penetrates from behind. Your G-spot receives an orgasmic massage, and he gets a titillating view of your bum.
SECRET TIP: *Try stepping out of the shower for your climax scene. My best bathroom poses are bending over and hanging on to the sink (great for eye contact in the mirror) and him sitting on the closed toilet lid with me straddling him.*

SECRET CONFESSIONS

Dressing up

I'm a recent convert to corsets. I love the way they mould my body into a perfect curvy shape and push my breasts up to make me look super-voluptuous. They change the way I act in bed, too – more brazen, more confident and more in charge. And, as I discovered, I'm not alone ...

"My boyfriend bought me a chambermaid outfit. It's brilliant! He can't take his eyes off me when I put it on. I do the classic chambermaid routine of dropping something, then slowly bending over in front of him so he can see my crotch outlined by my panties. I tie him up with a feather boa, too. It's great because normally I'm pretty reserved."

"I went to a fancy dress party with an erotic theme and dressed up in this amazing catsuit. It was black latex. It was so skin-tight it left nothing to the imagination. I'm happy to say that evening restored all my sexual confidence – I could just see the lust in people's eyes."

"It's not very risqué, but my favourite sexy outfit is a satin Japanese kimono that just about covers my bum. Underneath I wear a gorgeous pair of crotchless lace briefs and nothing else. It makes me feel incredibly feminine. My biggest turn on is watching his face as I stand by the bed and let the kimono slip from my body."

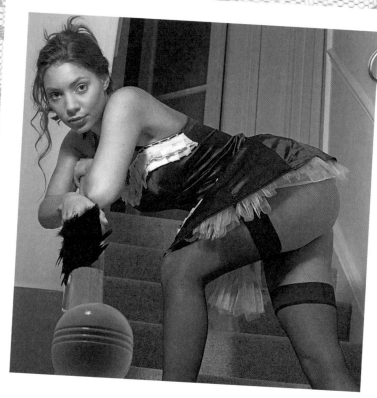

... A new persona

SECRET EROTIC TOYS

A friend of mine once told me she'd never bought a sex toy because she was so good at improvizing with household objects. This got me thinking. After our conversation I went home and started looking at my electric toothbrush in a whole new light! Then I noticed all the other everyday objects that I could repurpose for erotic pleasure. All it takes is a slightly kinky imagination.

BE A DOMESTIC SEX GODDESS

Try taking a tour of your house tonight – look for the sexual potential in ordinary items. Put anything that inspires you into a "toy box". It's thrilling to turn something ordinary into something erotic – and you and your lover can enjoy the secret pleasure that no-one will ever know. Here's my list of domestic sex toys:

- Rolling pin – A man's gluteal muscles can take a lot of pressure, and massaging his buttocks using a rolling-pin can feel a lot deeper and more satisfying than massage by hand. A furry paint roller can do the same job, with the advantage that he can return the favour by rolling it softly over your belly and breasts.
- An apron – make him breakfast in bed and take it to him dressed in just an apron. Then walk around giving him a sexy view of your bare back and bum.
- Exercise balls – try having sex on one. It's wobbly and precarious, but great fun. Ask him to straddle the ball, then sit on his lap and bounce.
- Beanbags – I discovered all sorts of sex positions feel fantastic on a beanbag because the tiny balls mould to the contours of your body. A great one is to lie on top on your tummy and then get your lover to enter you from behind.
- Oil drizzler – try this sensual treat. Empty out the olive oil from an oil drizzler and replace it with sweet-smelling coconut oil. Plunge the whole thing into a sink of very hot water and within 10 minutes it'll be ready to drizzle over your lover's naked body.

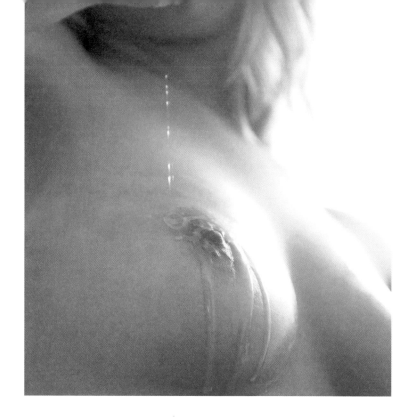

- A feather duster – it goes without saying: use it to tickle and polish him from head to toe, then he can return the favour.
- String of pearls/beads – ask him to unclasp them from your neck at the end of an evening, then take them from him and wind them seductively around his penis. If you want to improvize a clitoral stimulator during sex, leave them wrapped around the base of his penis as you climb on top.
- A stand-alone mirror – one night we tried picking ours up and laying it flat on the floor. Then we had sex astride it. It gave both of us an incredibly titillating view.
- Clothes pegs – if you want to make each other gasp, clothes pegs are the perfect alternative to nipple clamps. Take turns to put them on each other. Experiment with mild pain on other body parts, too – start with fleshy places such as the earlobes.
- Hair scrunchie – if you have long hair, keep it secured in a scrunchie all day, then whip it off at night to let your hair tumble around your shoulders. Now give him an erection and wind the scrunchie around the base of his penis. It'll act as an impromptu penis ring, helping to trap blood inside his penis (but don't make it too tight).

RAUNCHY ROLEPLAY

Whenever I'm in the mood for something exciting, I try roleplaying. There's something amazingly erotic about pretending to be someone else, plus it means I can do things that ordinarily would make me blush. Try roleplaying when you're in the mood for a sexual adventure. Start by asking yourself who you want to become; and how far you'll go to bring your role to life.

WHO WILL YOU BE TONIGHT?

Roleplaying can be light-hearted and frivolous or used to explore your deepest, darkest desires. On the light-hearted side, you could act out a fantasy between two strangers at a masked ball. On the darker side, you could play master and slave games. How far you go is up to you.

Most roleplaying games involve a difference in power – that's what gives roleplay its special frisson – so, if you're new to roleplaying, sit down with your lover and answer these questions (do this separately, then compare your answers):

+ Do you fantasize about being in charge and having complete sexual control?
+ If you're in charge, would you be kind and giving, or bossy and strict?
+ Do you fantasize about being helpless in bed?
+ If you'd like to be helpless, do you like the idea of being overpowered or "taken"?
+ Do you want to play different roles depending on your mood – sometimes dominant, sometimes submissive?

Now talk to your lover about how your fantasies could fit together. Does one of you want submission and the other dominance, or do you both crave either one? How do you feel about overpowering each other? Personally, I like to take turns depending on my mood. Let the conversation get steamy. When you're both feeling hot, discuss which of the following scenarios you'd like to try. All the roles are interchangeable – you just need to decide who takes the position of power.

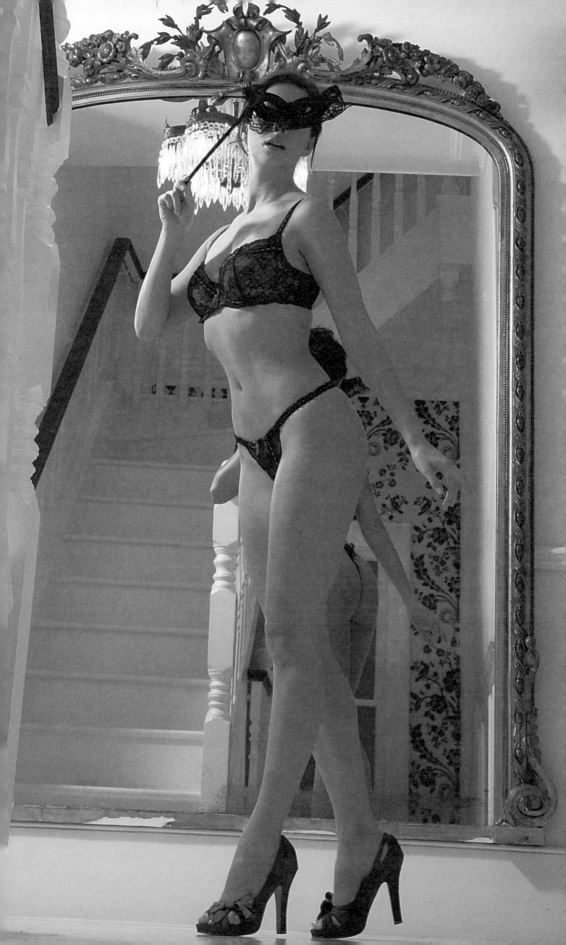

- Voyeur and exhibitionist – you're in your bedroom, taking your clothes off, caressing yourself. When you're naked and turned on, you start masturbating. Outside the bedroom door is a stranger who's been spying on you. He's extremely excited – what happens next?

- Sex therapist and client: you're visiting a sex therapist and it's his job to make you come using different methods. For professional reasons he can't indulge his own lust. Will you force him to misbehave?

- Boss and employee: you're the boss and working late with your employee. You start asking him to do increasingly intimate jobs from taking your shoes off, to massaging your feet, to undressing. He must carry out the jobs willingly and ask for nothing. When he's granted all your sexual requests, you have to decide whether to reward him.

- Escort and client: you've sought the services of a male escort for one night only. He's happy to do anything. Before you take your clothes off and get started, he questions you about your favourite sexual acts.

- Slave and master: you've been naughty and need discipline. Your master's job is to deliver erotic "punishment", such as spanking. If you're good, he'll reward you with oral sex or other sexual treats.

- Artist and model: the artist insists that you pose naked for him. You enjoy the eroticism of lying back knowing that every curve of your body is being observed and enjoyed.

SUBMISSIVE OR DOMINANT?

Women who have lots of responsibility, pressure and commitment in their life tell me they find it liberating to be helplessly dominated during sex – to finally let go and let someone else be boss. But if you're shy and retiring, you may find it exciting to let your powerful and commanding side out to play.

BRINGING THE ROLE TO LIFE

If roleplay is your thing, there are several ways of getting into character. Read this list with your lover and choose which techniques you'd most like to try.

+ Clothes – dressing up is great fun and can transform you. Whether you're exchanging some boring cotton panties for a lacy black thong, or he's slipping into a cop uniform, you'll definitely change your behaviour when you're dressed differently. A friend of mine has a special drawer dedicated to her "dressing-up" clothes.

+ Shoes – the right footwear may be all you need to propel you into a sexy role. For you it could be a simple pair of heels or some boots that make your legs look stunning. For him, it could be a sexy pair of cowboy boots.

+ Masks – not being able to see each other's faces by wearing a mask frees your imagination. (Fancy dress masks can be creepy so try wearing masquerade or Venetian masks.)

+ Blindfolds – if I can't see, I've always found it a lot easier to throw away my inhibitions (see pages 76–7).

+ Toys and props – as well as adding authenticity to your role, you can use toys and props to deliver pleasure and punishment to your lover. For example, no dominatrix is complete without a riding crop; no policewoman could manage without handcuffs; and no sex therapist could work without a range of sex toys to get to the bottom of her client's problems.

+ Voice and manner – if I'm playing a dominant role, I speak in a self-assured and commanding voice and tell my lover exactly what I'm going to do to him. If I'm in a submissive role, I speak in a soft, compliant voice and make it clear that I'll completely surrender to my lover's every wish.

SECRET TIP: *When I'm playing the dominant role, I unsettle my lover by being alternately loving and strict. I always find that unpredictability is incredibly erotic.*

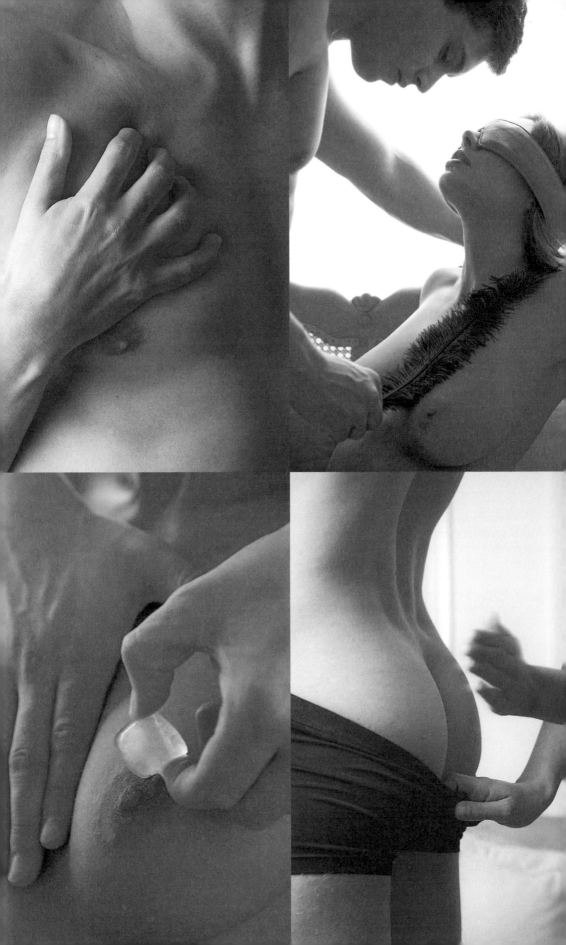

SECRETS OF ...

Pleasure and pain

+ **BE AN ICE QUEEN** Get him to smooth an ice cube around your nipples or your labia, clitoris and vagina. Afterwards he can make you melt by dripping warm (but not hot) water directly onto your clitoris. Or he can lick you after taking a sip of hot tea. True ice queens can go a step further: get him to caress you internally with an ice dildo (made using a lolly mould). Let it partially melt so you don't get frostbite.

+ **GIVE HIM GLOVE LOVE** Blindfold him, lay him flat on his black and then stroke his erect penis with different types of glove. Try a leather glove, a rubber glove, a woollen mitten or – my personal favourite – an elbow length silk glove. See which gets the most moans.

+ **PLAY WITH DIFFERENT SENSATIONS** Use feathers to stroke, fingernails to scratch or fingers to pinch. Take it in turns to wear a blindfold to heighten sensitivity.

+ **SPANK HIM** A pleasure my lover and I have recently discovered: softly caress his naked bum with your palm. Then give him two light taps followed by two hard spanks. Then go back to soft caresses. Always aim for the anal area – never the tailbone – and keep your hand slightly curved. Try these, too: spank him with the back of a hairbrush or a wooden spoon, or spank him through his jeans.

+ **GIVE HIM A HOT SURPRISE** Lay him down for a candlelit massage, then pick up the candle and use it to drip wax on him from the nape of his neck to the cleft of his buttocks. Rub the wax sensuously into his body. Caution: use only special "massage candles" (the wax melts at a lower temperature than normal candles).

SEX IN PUBLIC PLACES

If you've ever been aroused by the idea of having sex around other people, you're not alone. The idea of doing something naughty in public has always turned me on. But, as I've discovered, it's important to know how not to get caught in the act.

THE ART OF INVISIBILITY

Firstly, dress for the occasion. This means easily liftable skirts/dresses (and no panties) and easy access flies. One good tip: a boyfriend once advised me to dress in smart clothes because if you look formal or official, people are more likely to give you the benefit of the doubt.

Secondly, position is everything – arrange your bodies in a way that's as ambiguous as possible. I once had a fantastic afternoon in a park while curled up in a spoons position under a blanket. I've also sat on my lover's lap for a "cuddle" on a secluded bench and wrapped my legs around his waist for a romp in the sea.

Thirdly, rather than attempting the in and out thrusts of intercourse, have internal, Tantric-style sex that relies on vaginal squeezes and penile flexes. Even if it doesn't give you an orgasm, you'll feel incredibly naughty, and you can carry on at home later. If you can't resist up and down movements, make them slow and infrequent. Or for my tips on how to have sex in minutes, see pages 106–109.

THE PRIVATE ALTERNATIVE TO GOING PUBLIC

If public sex is too risky, try this: have sex in front of a window, but without being obviously visible. You'll still get the "someone-could-see-us" thrills, but without the risk of arrest. Try any of these tricks: make the room as dark as possible during the day and position a chair a short way from the window. Or have sex in front of a high hotel room window or a low basement window. Turn each other on with words – now's the time to use all your dirty talk skills. If I'm in a public place where I can be overheard, I use codewords for the saucy bits.

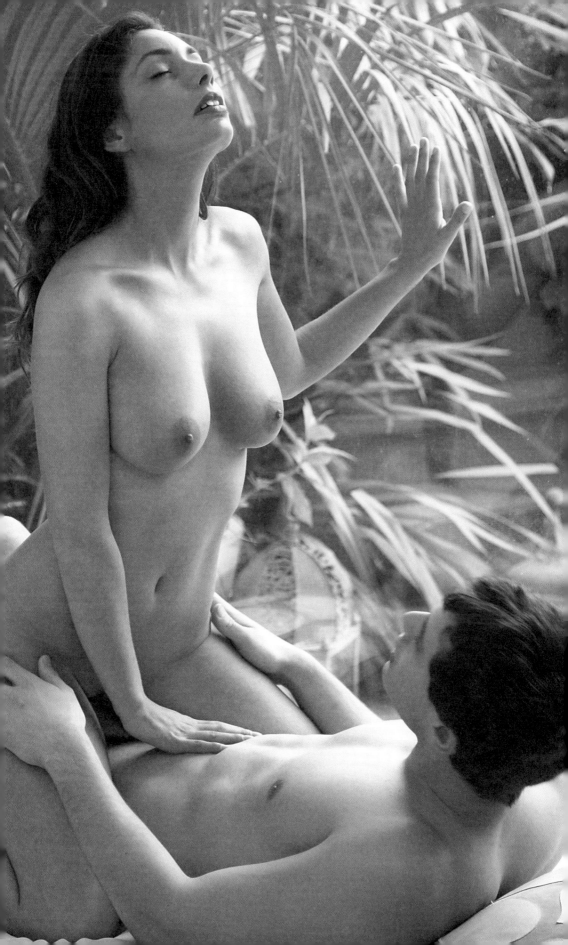

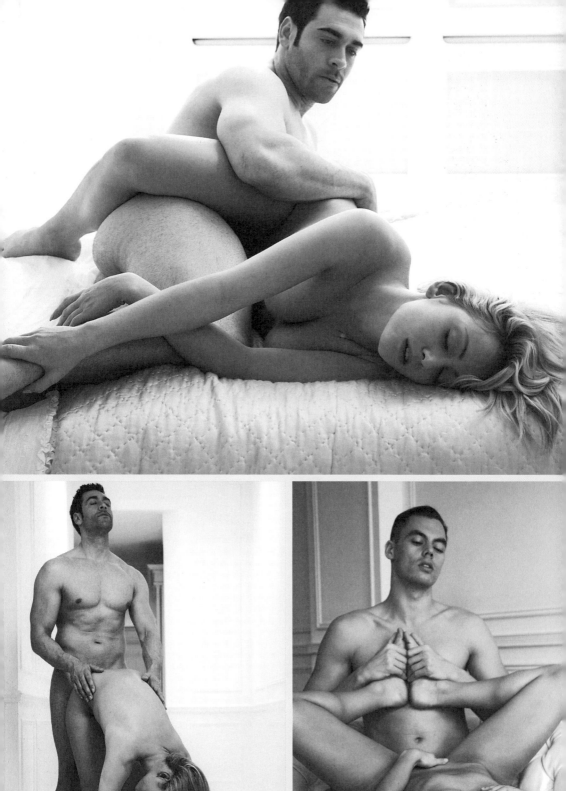

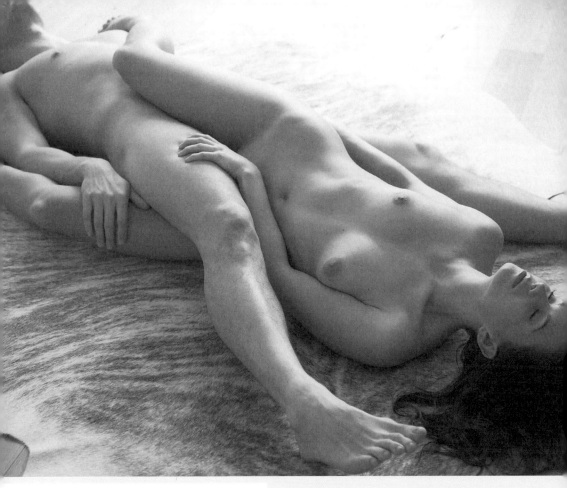

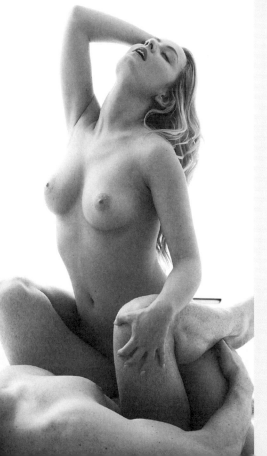

ADVANCED SEX POSITIONS

TRY ANY OF THESE WHEN YOU'RE IN THE MOOD FOR A CHALLENGE. Novel angles and positions can make sex feel exciting and experimental. You may even discover hotspots you didn't know you had. Even physically demanding postures, such as bending forward to touch the floor, are worth it for the psychological thrill. Often, for him, it's all about the view. If he can look down and gaze at your bum or breasts, he'll be more than happy.

HOW TO DO AN EROTIC DANCE

I used to think erotic dancing should be left to professional dancers. After all, there was no way I could compete with a trained pole dancer. Then I discovered that lots of private dance studios offer workshops in pole dancing, can-can and burlesque – not just for professionals, but for anyone. So I went along with a friend. As well as being great fun (and an excellent workout), my lover was delighted with the results when I danced for him at home.

Dancing for your lover is an amazing experience – as well as taking him to a peak of excitement, you'll get drunk on erotic power. You don't have to be a great dancer – you just have to discover your inner diva and embrace her with open arms.

GETTING INTO CHARACTER

Slipping into a costume is a great way to get in the mood. Try:

+ Burlesque – dress in corset, fishnets, suspenders, beads, feather boa, elbow-length gloves and a hat with a veil.
+ Fetish – wear a PVC basque and killer heels or thigh-high boots.
+ Glamorous – keep it skimpy but stunning: your most gorgeous bra (or nipple tassels) and panties.
+ Fantasy – dress up as your, or his, favourite fantasy: nurse, maid, bunny girl, cop or waitress.
+ Next to nothing – adopt the less-is-more principle. Try a thong and pasties (adhesive nipple covers), or hold-up stockings and a bow tie.

SECRET TIP: *If you're shy, invent a version of yourself that's braver, sassier and more brazen. Professional erotic dancers dream up a fantasy of themselves, then take that fantasy on stage.*

THE MOVES

I was taught the following classic erotic dance moves – you'll need a chair with no arms that you can pick up easily. You'll also need to be able to swing your leg over the back. Enjoy practising the moves in front of a mirror. Alternatively, do what I did: next time you want to have a party with some female friends, make it a "teach yourself erotic dancing party". It's a great way to have a laugh and get some feedback.

Start by positioning your chair facing your audience/partner. Now stand a couple of steps behind it, close your eyes and immerse yourself in the opening notes of the music …

1 Stand with your legs apart and hold onto the back of your chair. Lean forward to show lots of sexy cleavage. Start swirling your hips in large slow circles or figures of eight. Tips: keep bending your knees in time with your moves. Keep your back straight and your head up.

2 Strut sexily from the back of the chair to the front – take high steps and place each foot exactly in front of the other foot, swaying your hips provocatively as you go. Tips: leave one hand on the back of the chair as you strut and, to sit down, place your feet wide apart, keep your back straight and sway your hips from side to side until your bum meets the seat.

3 Sit on the seat of the chair with your thighs pressed together. Slip your fingers between the tops of your thighs and then slide them down your legs "forcing" them apart until they're in a provocative, wide-open "V" position. Tip: keep only your tiptoes on the floor – it elongates your calves.

4 With your legs still wide apart and your hands resting on the top of your thighs, move your hips in circles (imagine you're trying to spin a hoop very slowly while sitting down). Slide your hands up your thighs and over the front of your body. Keep the hip circles going. If your hair is long enough, push it on top of your head and let it tumble sexily down again. Tip: let the circular moves from your hips radiate up your body so that your chest and shoulders move, too.

5 Swivel on your chair by 45 degrees so you're sitting side on. Keep your legs together. Grip the edge of the seat behind you. Thrust your breasts forward and arch your back (so your buttocks lift off the seat slightly). Now rock backward and forward on your seat. Push your breasts out as far as you can on each forward movement. Tip: enjoy the sexiness of the movement – close your eyes and turn your head slightly to the side.

6 Move to the edge of the seat. Keep rocking but make it incredibly slow. On a backward rock, lean back more than usual and raise one straight leg seductively in the air. If you can, point your toe to the ceiling. Lower your leg. On the next backward rock raise the other leg. Keep doing this. Tip: this looks incredible when it's done slowly and effortlessly (so work on your leg muscles). Also by going super-slow you're letting him know you're in charge. If you find yourself rushing, count one … two … three … four … slowly in your head.

7 Now swing one leg over the back of the chair so you're straddling the seat with your back to your lover. Grip the back of the chair with your hands and do the slow spin-a-hoop move you did in step 4. Again, get your chest and shoulders in on the act. Tip: keep changing the direction of your hip circles.

8 Stop circling your hips and slowly get up so you're in a standing strad-dle. Take hold of the back of the seat and pull it out from between your legs. Turn the chair round so you can grip the back. Take a few steps back until you're bending over almost at right angles. Now move your bum in circles or figures of eight (as you did in step 1). Tip: push your bum as high in the air as you can.

9 Slowly stand up and turn to face your lover Strut sexily toward him, then straddle him so that your breasts are positioned tantalizingly close to his face. At this point you can either abandon yourselves to lust or you can pull back and tease him with more dancing. Remember – you're in control.

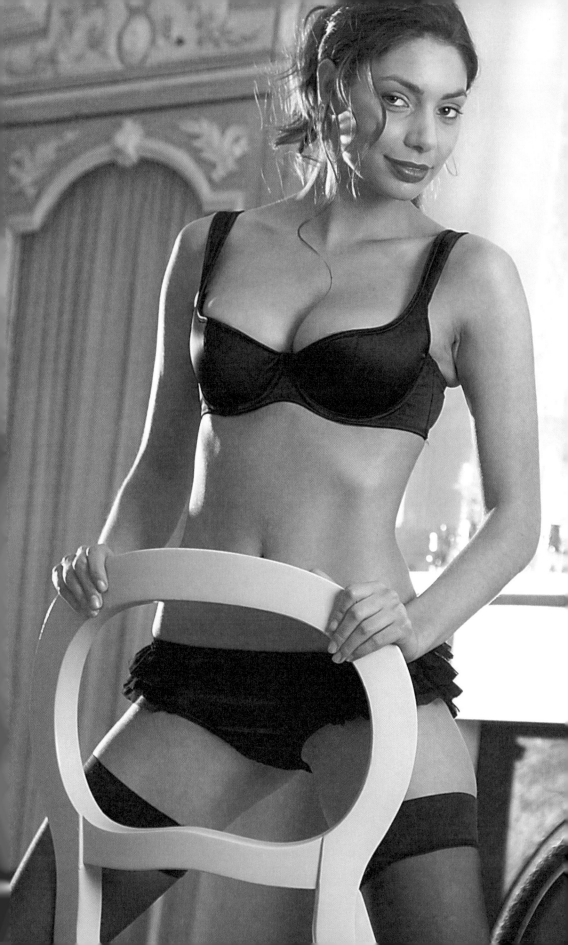

SEXY BONDAGE TECHNIQUES

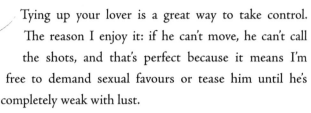

Tying up your lover is a great way to take control. The reason I enjoy it: if he can't move, he can't call the shots, and that's perfect because it means I'm free to demand sexual favours or tease him until he's completely weak with lust.

SECRET TIP: *I've noticed that men are reluctant to admit they like the vulnerability of being tied up. Yet once they're bound to the bed they find it incredibly erotic. Take the lead – tell him you're doing it for your own pleasure rather than his.*

GATHER YOUR PROPS

Most people think of ropes and handcuffs when they think of bondage, but unless you want to engage in serious kinkiness, these are some of the friendlier options for making your lover into a sexy captive.

+ Silk scarves – these are great because they can serve a dual purpose. After you've wafted them seductively over your lover's body, in particular his penis, balls and belly, you can use them to tie his ankles and wrists to the bed. Just don't tie silk scarves too tight (and keep a pair of scissors handy in case the knots are difficult to undo).

+ Bondage tape – it might sound daunting, but bondage tape is one of the simplest and safest types of restraint (great for beginners). It's like sticky tape, except it comes in more exciting colours, it's satisfyingly stretchy and as it only sticks to itself, it's completely painless when removed (no unintended waxing). The first time you use it, wrap it around your captive's ankles or wrists.

+ Velcro cuffs – things have come a long way from hard-core metal handcuffs. You can find fur-lined cuffs with quick-release Velcro fastenings in any online sex shop. They're quick and easy to slap on him when he's been naughty and they won't cut off his blood supply.

+ Spank ties – these bendy toys are perfect for novices. They're lengths of flexible metal coated in comfortably soft rubber. As well as being easy to use, they're surprisingly versatile. They can be used to give your lover a naughty spank, before tying him up.

SECRET TIP: Try making love in a sex sling (you can buy them in online sex shops). They pull your legs high into the air as you lie on your back. They give both of you deliciously taut sensations.

GETTING INTO A BIND

The most popular position for being tied up is lying spread-eagled on the bed. It's a bondage cliché, but it's got a lot to recommend it: it leaves the captive's genitals exposed, which provides intense erotic vulnerability, and easy access to hotspots; and because the captive's arms are secured, there's no choice but to surrender. It's the ultimate in sexual submission and highly arousing for those who enjoy domination.

RULES OF ENGAGEMENT
Even if you're only doing some light dabbling in the world of bondage, follow these safety guidelines:
- *Agree a codeword that means "stop, I've had enough". Always choose something other than the word "stop" because shouting this is often part of the fun.*
- *Don't tie him up and leave him on his own.*
- *Don't tie anything around the neck, and don't cut off circulation – you should always be able to slide one or two fingers between your lover's skin and the restraint.*

SEX SECRETS

When you're tired of the spread-eagled position, try some of the
following lesser-known tricks:

+ Get him to bind your knees together. The benefit is that it pulls your
  thighs tightly together and ensures an extremely snug fit when he
  climbs on top and tries to penetrate you. Either that or he'll have to
  help you onto your knees and enter you from behind. Bondage tape
  is the best type of tool for binding the knees – don't use a silk scarf
  because as soon as you wiggle your legs, it will slip down.
+ Take it in turns to bind each other's body in cling film (although a
  quick safety note: do this only below the neck; and leave the arms
  free). When your lover is the bound one, tease him by kissing him
  passionately and flicking your tongue against his shrink-wrapped
  penis and testicles. His tightly trapped erection will be a huge turn-
  on for both of you.
+ When tying your lover's hands together, instead of binding his wrists
  with the palms face to face, tell him to cross his wrists in front of his
  body, then wrap a long, skinny scarf around them in a criss-cross
  fashion. This not only looks sexier, it also allows him to put his arms
  behind his head while you have your wicked way with him. Let him
  do the same to you.
+ Try this Japanese technique – get him to rest his forearms in the
  small of his back (so he clasps the opposite elbow with each hand).
  Now bind his arms.
+ Immobilize him quickly by tying his arms to his legs. Simply ask him
  to relax his arms by his sides. Then wind bondage tape or a spank tie
  all the way around his right wrist and his right thigh. Repeat on the
  left side, and he's all yours.
+ Ask him to make you a "dress" by winding bondage tape round and
  round your body from your chest to your thighs (leaving your arms
  free). Tell him to leave gaps in the tape to give him tongue access to
  your nipples and clitoris.

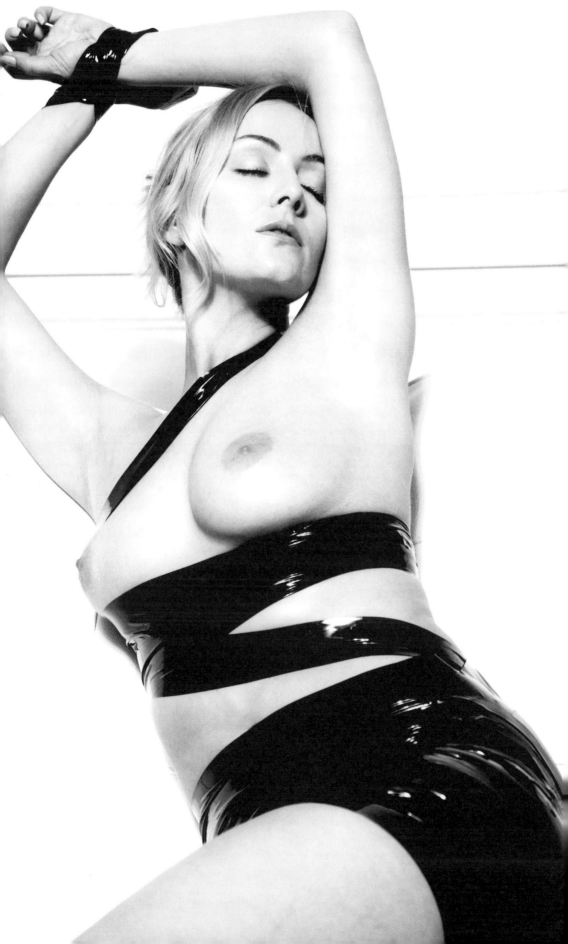

SHOOT YOUR OWN EROTICA

A naughty film is fun to make, but it's even more thrilling to watch back later. "Home videos" are my favourite adult viewing – they kick-start sex when I watch them with my lover. And casting myself as a sex star does amazing things for my sexual confidence.

Before you start, promise that anything you create will only be seen by each other. Or, if it makes you more comfortable, watch the footage once, then delete it from the camera. Men love X-rated surprises. I once made a secret video of myself having a very sexy shower. I packed it in my lover's suitcase as a surprise present when he went away on business.

Make the preparation for filming part of the fun. Have a shower together and kiss while you're soaping each other. Then slip into some sexy underwear, turn the heating up and prepare your movie set. Follow the tips on page 62 for making a love nest, but instead of using candles, keep the room well lit. Flirt and touch each other. Rub baby oil into each other's skin so you both look gorgeously strokable on camera.

SECRET TIP: *Get really intimate: discuss what pubic hairstyle would look sexy for your starring role, then take it turns to shave or trim each other.*

OPENING SHOTS

Now you've prepared yourselves and your room, it's time to shoot the opening scene to your movie. This is your chance for some playful exhibitionism. Ask your lover to hand-hold the camera (beckon him over if you want him to film a close up). Any of the following scenes make a provocative beginning:

- You seductively removing your stockings and panties while looking into the camera.
- A tour of your body by camera (your lover provides a sexy commentary and gives you instructions about you how he'd like you

to stand, sit or lie). Flirt with your lover as he films you. Or play coy by covering your breasts/genitals at first and then gradually revealing more as you get "braver".

+ You lying on the bed caressing yourself while your lover "interviews" you about your favourite sexual acts. (Watch the film *Sex, Lies and Videotape* for inspiration.)

+ You massaging body oil into your skin and getting more and more steamed up.

+ You and your lover standing in front of a full-length mirror having a conversation about what you're going to do. When the discussion gets really X-rated, take turns to hold the camera while you give each other oral sex.

Shooting one of these opening scenes acts as full-on foreplay, so you'll probably be smouldering in a matter of minutes. When you can't take any more, ask him to fix the camera on a tripod/nearby surface, check that the whole of your body (plus a surrounding area of bed) appears in the frame, then press "record".

CLOSER THAN CLOSE

If you want to create an erotic video with a different mood and feel from one shot on a tripod-mounted camera, take turns to hold the camera by hand while you have sex. The result will feel more intimate because of the extremely close range. You can capture incredibly personal details, for example, his penis penetrating you or his expression of orgasmic bliss. The main drawbacks are that your framing won't be perfect or the camera will jiggle when you're at the height of passion. And there's a danger of dropping the camera when things really hot up ...

THE XXX ACTION

Once you've beckoned him over and pulled him on top of you, all you need to do is go wild and let the camera capture your lust. When you're in the throes of passion, try to remember at least some of these secrets of on-camera sex:

+ Do a bit of everything: he goes down on you, you go down on him, then when you have sex, keep switching positions, or have a break for more oral sex, hand caresses or mutual masturbation.
+ Include sex toys to keep the action varied.
+ Make sure you both climax – it's exciting to watch at playback time.
+ Make your thrusts, grinds and wriggles big and dramatic –prolonged small movements may feel great, but they aren't so exciting to look back on when you're viewing your footage.
+ Don't keep looking at the camera to check it's recording – immerse yourself in the action.
+ Don't get so immersed in your lovemaking that you forget the camera and roll out of range.
+ Connect your camera to a television so you can see what you're filming while you're filming it. Seeing the action unfold not only allows you to check you're in the frame, it also sends your arousal levels sky-high.

YOUR FUTURE IN FILM

If you enjoyed filming yourselves, try doing it again with a twist: instead of shooting everyday sex, try shooting one of the roleplaying scenarios on pages 130–132. Dress up, write a film-script and speak in character. It doesn't matter if the plot is thin, you'll still have lots of sexy giggles before, during and after.

If you want to add a more professional touch to any erotic video, try taking different bits of footage and interspersing close-ups with longer-range shots.

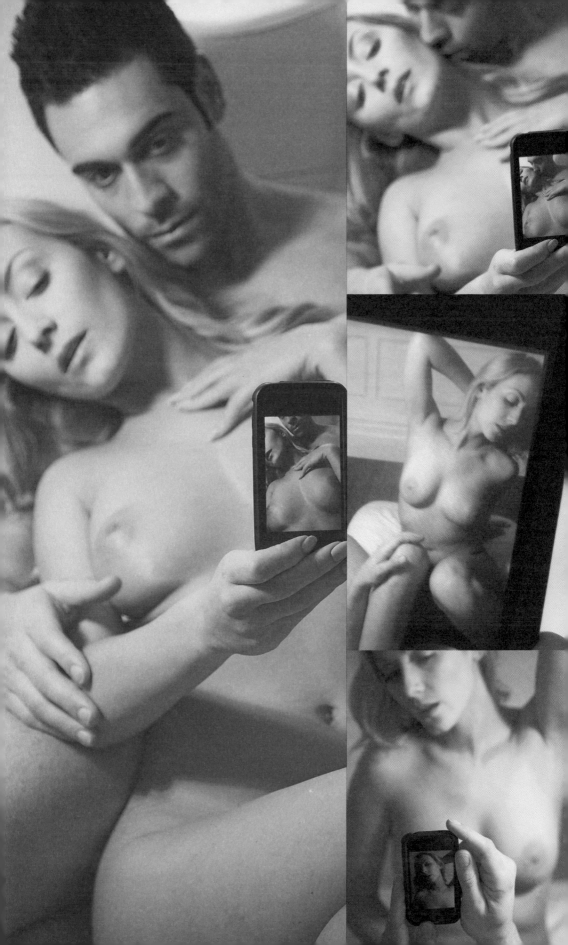

SECRET CONFESSIONS
Spanking

I had an exciting evening of spanking recently. Not the dress-up-as-a-schoolgirl type of spanking – more a massage that turned naughty. I'd just given my lover a back rub and was finishing off with some strong hacking strokes. I noticed that everytime I hit his bum his moans got louder. So instead of using the sides of my hands, I started spanking him with the flats of my hands instead. He loved it.

I asked him to do it back to me and I found it not just erotic, but surprisingly sensual. It seems spanking is popular with lots of people ...

"My partner sometimes spanks me during sex. It sends a shock wave of pleasure up my body and makes me gasp. I like the fact that I never know when he's going to do it."

"We discovered spanking when we were play-fighting. I was pretending to be really angry with him. I pulled his trousers off and began spanking him. I started getting really into it and couldn't stop! He got really turned on."

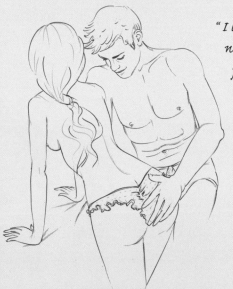

" I love the stinging sensation on my bum. It's not pain exactly. More like a hot tingling feeling. I like it when he follows it up with a nice gentle massage, too."

"I'm a traditionalist. I like bending over with my hands on my knees. And my lover has to tell me off while he's spanking me. That's the bit I find most erotic."

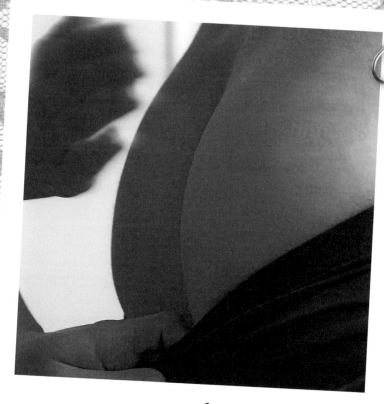

... *So naughty*

DIRTY WEEKEND

When I haven't had any quality time with my lover, the best way I know to reconnect is a weekend away. It's a perfect recipe for sexiness: two uninterrupted days in bed; unfamiliar surroundings; a bottle of wine chilling by the bedside; and room service just a call away.

Dirty weekends can invigorate your sex life – the erotic after-glow stays with you for days, plus you'll feel fantastically naughty, and deeply connected with your lover. Perhaps the best part is that you've got rid of everyday distractions – so you can shed your inhibitions and try those sexy acts you've fantasized about.

BEFORE YOU GO

Propose the idea of a dirty weekend to your lover over dinner one night. Promise him two days – and nights – of pure pleasure and sexy treats – no pressure to do anything except have fun.

I try to take as little as possible with me when I go away with my lover – and only sensual or sexy items. Include any of these in your weekend bag: thongs, stockings, basque, blindfold, massage oil, feathers, condoms, silk bathrobe, sexy dress, erotic novel, perfume, candles, iPod loaded with sexy music.

SECRET TIP: *Men love surprises that cater specifically to their sexual tastes. For example, if blowjobs are his thing, he'll be delighted if you pull out some edible lube from your suitcase and offer to apply it.*

DAY 1

When you arrive at your destination, start as you mean to go on – go straight to bed. Have a salacious chat about the room's erotic potential. Plan to get frisky in various places: up against the door, in the shower, in an armchair, in front of a window or mirror, and on the balcony or in the pool. You could even find out whether you can get onto the roof for some surreptitious love beneath the stars.

Treat everything that happens from now on as foreplay – even if you have a shower, make it slow, luxurious and steeped in eroticism. Invite your lover to join you or to wrap you up in a towel as you emerge all steamy and wet.

Discover each other's naked bodies beneath or on top of the sheets. Taste each other's lips. Tour his body with your tongue. Give each other a long full-body massage and lingering kisses. Be aware of all the tingling, fizzing, throbbing or warm feelings building up inside you. Don't act on them – yet.

When you couldn't be any more aroused, take it in turns to ask each other for sexual favours. When it's your turn, describe what you want in lascivious detail. For example, if you want oral sex, say where you want it (for example, "sitting on the chair by the desk"), how you want it (for example, "lots of slow licks on my clitoris") and what you want to happen next (for example, "pick me up and carry me to bed").

Make this erotic turn-taking the theme for the whole day. Include it in everything you do, even the things that aren't explicitly sexual, for example, "I'd like you to feed me dinner".

Wait until nighttime to have explosive sex that leaves you totally exhausted in each other's arms.

SECRET TIP: *A dirty weekend is a great time to introduce him to a new sex toy – both of you will be feeling relaxed and experimental.*

DAY 2

Devote today to trying things you've never tried before. Create some red-hot memories. Here are some ideas to inspire you:

+ Render him completely helpless by blindfolding him in a dark room and binding his wrists and ankles. Put earphones into his ears and play him some sexy music. Now "torture" him with sexual treats.

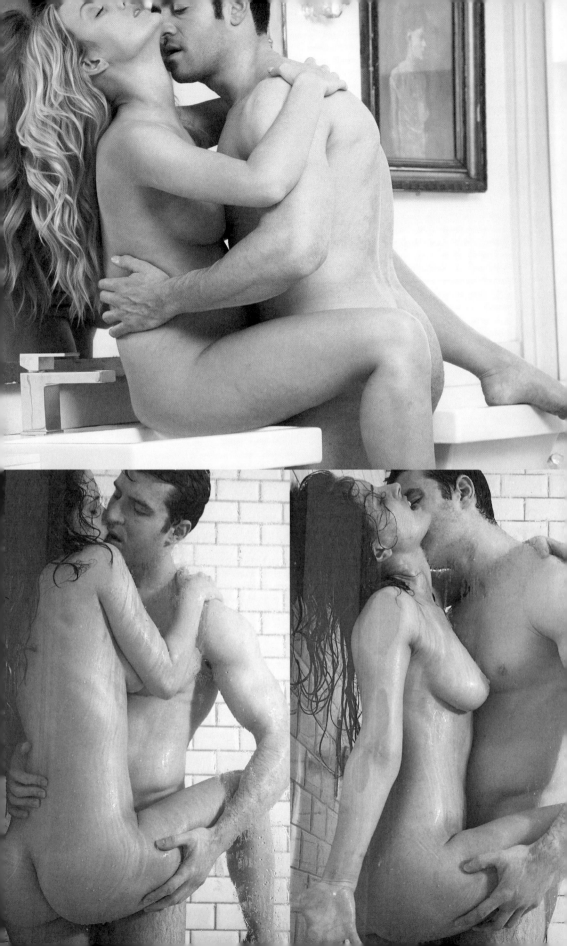

- Try some Japanese-style sex play (advance preparation needed). For example, decorate his penis with origami (look up *kokigami* on the internet) or get him to arrange sushi on your body (look up *nyotaimori*). Alternatively, try playing with eggs. Break two eggs and separate the yolks from the whites. After he's swallowed the yolks whole or slipped them into your mouth from his (not to everyone's taste!), he rubs the slippery egg whites into your inner thighs and genitals. This is an old Japanese ritual that was used to prepare a virgin for sex (over the course of seven nights the man wiggled his lubricated fingers a little deeper into her vagina).
- Explore the fetish world of "WAM" (wet and messy). Cover the floor with sheets or towels and wrestle, wriggle and writhe together while covered in a slick, wet, slippery substance such as oil, cream, body lotion or honey.
- Try body painting – it's a sexy way to become intimate with your lover's body and him with yours. It's also erotic and relaxing to feel gentle brush strokes tickling your hotspots. You can use face paint (or edible body paint if you plan to lick your lover clean afterwards). Ask him to paint swirls along your thighs. Tease him by painting your name on the shaft of his penis. Look on the internet for some inspirational whole-body painting techniques.
- Take advantage of the fact that you're in a hotel room – dress up as a kinky chambermaid and treat him to a teasing roleplay. Address him only as "sir".
- Take it in turns to give each other a genital massage for at least 20 minutes. When it's your turn to massage him, use long, sweeping, exploratory strokes that don't lead him straight to orgasm.
- Try disappearing from the hotel room for long enough to make your lover concerned, then send him a text telling him to come to the hotel bar. Throw yourselves into a strangers-meeting-for-the-first-time roleplay.

LEARN MORE ...

As I was writing *Sex Secrets*, I came across a huge amount of sexy information. Here are just a few books and websites that I'd like to share with you.

When you feel like going to bed and snuggling up with an erotic book, try these: (If your lover is in bed with you, read aloud to him.)

* Agent Provocateur *Confessions* (Pavilion Books, 2006)
* Agent Provocateur *V, The Secret Life of V* (Pavilion Books, 2007)
* Blue, Violet *Lust* (Cleis Press, 2007)
* Blue, Violet *Sweet Life: Erotic Fantasies for Couples* (Cleis Press, 2001)
* Blue, Violet *In Bed With ...* (Sphere, 2008)
* Blue, Violet *Best Women's Erotica 2010* (Cleis Press, 2001)
* *The New Erotic Photography* (Taschen, 2009)

Or for something more informative that might just increase your sexpertise:

* Anand, Margot *The New Art of Sexual Ecstasy* (Thorsons, 2003)
* Chalker, Rebecca *The Clitoral Truth* (Seven Stories Press, 2000)
* Douglass, Marcia *Are We Having Fun Yet? The Intelligent Woman's Guide to Sex* (Little, Brown and Company, 1997)
* Hite, Shere *The New Hite Report* (Octopus, 2000)
* Royalle, Candida *How to Tell a Naked Man What to Do: Sex Advice from a Woman Who Knows* (Piatkus, 2006)

If you're in the mood for browsing gorgeous lingerie and sexy toys, try any of these sites:

* www.agentprovocateur.com
* www.coco-de-mer.com
* www.jimmyjane.com
* www.myla.com

And for some sexy reading online:

* www.emandlo.com
* www.erotica-uk.com
* www.scarletmagazine.co.uk

And if you'd like to look at my website:

* www.nicolebailey.co.uk

INDEX

AUTHOR'S ACKNOWLEDGMENTS
Thanks to Grace Cheetham and Manisha Patel at Duncan Baird Publishers, and Dawn Bates, Emma Forge and Tom Forge.

PUBLISHER'S ACKNOWLEDGMENTS
The publisher would like to thank:
Photography: John Davies, except for the lace image: Deborah Wolfe/iStockphoto
Photographic assistant: Dave Foster
Illustrations: Susie Hogarth
Make-up artist: Alli Williams
Models: supplied by International Models Management (IMM), Needhams Models and Target Models.